RATIONAL FASTING

A SCIENTIFIC METHOD OF FASTING YOUR WAY TO HEALTH

ARNOLD EHRET

Translated from the German
"KRANKE MENSCHEN"
by Dr. Benedict Lust M.D., N.D., D.O.
and edited by John B. Lust

Benedict Lust Publications, New York, N.Y. 10016

Rational Fasting
©Copyright *1971*
by Benedict Lust Publications
Library of Congress Catalog Number 72-125413
A BENEFICIAL BOOK Edition

First printing ....October, 1971
Second printing ....March, 1977

This *Beneficial Book* edition includes all the text of Arnold Ehret's original
and basic hard cover book, *Kranke Menschen*, published 1914 in
Munich, Germany. It is printed from brand new plates made from completely
reset, clear, easy-to-read type. *Beneficial Books* are published in pocket
book form by a division of Benedict Lust Publications, Box 404,
New York, N.Y. 10016

Contents

Contents (continued)

PART II

Introduction
by
Dr. Guy Bogart, N.D.

Are we booked, charted and checked for a return trip to the Garden of Eden? Is the fountain of youth to bubble forth in each man's front yard? Are we to forsake the soda fountain for the organized water of the unfermented grape? Are we to extract from the air our individual supply of nitrogen? Are bald pates to lose their aridity and to flourish with the effloresence of youth?

Professor Arnold Ehret, noted European savant, who spent his last years among Southern California's growing colony of celebrities, gives an affirmative answer to the above queries.

Toppling from the pedestals of traditionary superstition many of the old ideas of health, Professor Ehret gave more than a quarter of a century to intensive thinking and experimenting. He found the boasted white race but an aggregation of "corpse-colored" beings. More orthodox medical authorities have told us we are fast becoming a toothless race. Professor Ehret agreed with this finding and peeps along the pathway just a little farther to a "no-western-race-at-all" goal—

Unless—

Here comes the professor, not with any utopian

dreams, but with a carefully worked-out scheme of dietetic and health reform which some of the wisest doctors of two continents are hailing as the most fundamental word yet spoken in the complex maze of health panaceas. There is one unique feature of this expert's method of working—his experiments were uniformly conducted upon himself. In the fifteen years that he operated his big sanitarium in Switzerland, during his lectures and clinics in the biggest cities of Europe, and by thousands of consultations by post and telegraph in America and Europe, as well as practice in Asia and Africa during study trips, Professor Ehret had no lack of experience in observing results of his theories applied over a long period of time.

It was on his own person, however, that experiments were made before being tried out on patients. "Physician heal thyself" did not worry this wizard of the sanitarium, for he began his search while holding a professorship in a Badensian college, where he became "incurably" ill with Bright's disease. The complete restoration to health—to what was probably the most perfect state of health of anyone in our Western civilization today—and the adventure of finding the fundamental laws underlying the problems of life, liberty and the pursuit of health became a life work.

"Mucus" is the key-note of the attack which Ignorance has centered upon the Western civilization. A mucusless diet, coupled with a wise use of the fasting method, the whole adapted to the individual patient, but observing basic laws—confirmed by the physiological chemists and dietitians of some of the biggest universities—worked into a system of cure evolved entirely by Professor Ehret is the wand by which the toothless race is to be held back and western civilization given a new lease on life.

Most schools of healing have united on the idea that disease, regardless of its symptoms, consists of a constitutional encumbrance of a material generally known as foreign matter. Natural healing, consequently, consists of methods of treatment to eliminate this disease-producing material, and to stop the source of it. At least so reason a great number of the members of the healing profession; and it is the perfection of this idea that made Ehret a wizard among his kind.

My first knowledge of Professor Arnold Ehret came a few years ago when a translation of one of his important monographs came to my review desk. I was at once aroused, and, when he came to Los Angeles, was eager to make his acquaintance. Later I had the privilege of sitting through courses of lectures in his classes, of meeting him socially through a long period, of having his expert advice in my own dietetic practice, and of testing out to my own satisfaction the principles of health which he has discovered. It is from these sources that I shall try to set down, partly in his own language and partly in paraphrase, the story of the man and his record in the healing sphere. Only the broad outlines, of course, can be attempted, for while fundamentally simple, the Mucusless Diet Healing

System is a matter for more detailed study than can be covered here.

The general agreement on the part of at least the drugless healers and a large proportion of the medical fraternity that the fundamental cause of disease is the presence of foreign material in the body has not led to a basic discovery of the roots of this invading mystery. This material (and here and following I am speaking for Professor Ehret) is the undigested, uneliminated and decayed food elements from wrong and too-much eating. It is, consequently, most important, reasonable and clearly seen that the main factor in the health enigma should consist of dietetics, and this includes intelligently conducted fasting, especially if overeating is the main cause of the patient's disease. The method works the same in the human body as instinctive self-healing does in the animal.

The entire system is based upon Ehret's famous mucus theory, now a well-proven fact, and makes plain the former mysteries of all the 57 varieties of disease, including the "flu," pellagra and the jazz dance. The disease-producing material is a partially digested, decaying, semi-liquid mostly, and in this condition is generally known as mucus. It is easily proven and demonstrated that everyone living on a mixed diet (vegetables and meat), or a starchy vegetarian regimen, has a system more or less clogged up with mucus, whether sick or not. This foundation cause of every disease is going on from childhood and even before, if animal flesh and animal food products (fats) and starchy foods are eaten. It has long been recognized by students and scientists that these foods are not suitable for mankind, as the larger portion cannot be digested fully, but are acted on by the gastric juices making a toxic mucus which decays, ferments, produces gas, acidosis and many kinds of toxins; and this has a sticky, gluey consistency which clogs the circulation, so the body needs a shock like a "cold" to start the elimination of a portion of it.

If physical treatments are resorted to, they can eliminate only a portion as long as the supply is not stopped by a change from the mucus-forming foods and by overeating. It is reasonable, natural and self-evident, therefore, that the disease-producing eating must be stopped if you will have complete success from physical treatments.

Fasting and a decrease in the amount eaten is the only check on overeating, and non-mucus-forming foods must replace mucus-forming disease-producing ones. Professor Ehret did not invent or originate fasting or the use of fruit and green-leaf vegetables in improved diet, as these were recognized factors, but he did bring the greatest efficiency in their use by originating an entirely new system of combining them as a systematic healing method, under the name of The Mucusless Diet Healing System, after his "mucus theory" had become a well-proven fact as being the largest factor of the fundamental cause of every diseased condition.

Neither fasting nor fruit diet have been used in

strict accordance with the condition of the patient;
but to combine them as a "Systematic Cleansing"
the success is remarkable and satisfactory.

The greatest difference between a diet of Healing
and a diet of Nourishment is a point that needs
greatest emphasis. Fruit is the ideal practical and
natural diet of mankind, for nourishment, but the
mucusless diet is a regimen of healing and consists
of raw and cooked fruits, starchless and leafy
vegetables and mucus-poor cereals specially prepared. The ordinary diagnosis is not needed, nor
the local name of the disease; but the amount of
the encumbrance of mucus and the activity of the
toxins is of the first importance, and then the
degree to which the individual's encumbrance has
affected his vitality. Whether the patient is able to
labor and desires to do so, or whether he is more
seriously incapacitated determines the speed of
elimination, and upon this depends the degree of
weakness and disturbing sensations. For this cure is
the only one recorded which can be regulated and
controlled as to speed.

Action of the muscular and nerve systems is chemically lowered by the toxins of the mucus. To see
how these conditions affect the organic functions
and impair the vitality, in each individual case, is
the diagnosis.

It is an erroneous idea that only the blood is
affected, is unclean, full of mucus and toxins. The
entire body in its deepest tissues have these poisons
stored up. The amount of it is much more than is

supposed; consequently when it is dissolved and loosened by the mucusless diet, care must be taken not to do it too rapidly, for that clogs the excretory system, impairs the vital energy which is already weakened, and causes a serious condition. Even death may follow an unwise application of the eliminative process. This is important and explains why long fasts or fasts without proper preparation, and radical fruit cures often fail. Ehret's diagnosis is a conclusion from his knowledge of the aforementioned points, together with the general appearance of the patient, as to how rapidly he can stand the dissolving of his stored mucus, and then advises a transition diet that will make a gradual change from his mucus-forming foods to the full action of the mucusless diet. As soon as the greater part of the mucus "deposit" is dissolved and eliminated, a strict mucusless diet is advisable and if necessary can be combined with longer or shorter fasts depending upon the individual's condition.

In this cure, special attention is given to the bowel movements, as the intestines are the main organs of waste elimination. Artificial means can be used temporarily from above and below, but the mucusless diet is the only thorough and perfect cleanser that dissolves the dried mucus which sticks to the inner walls of the intestines and colon: and also furnishes the blood with the proper elements which dissolve the mucus that is stored up in the walls of the alimentary canal and which stops its peristalic action. To do this is the crowning action in the cure of constipation, something no other method of diet or any laxative has ever succeeded in doing.

The fruits of the mucusless diet furnish the blood with the best nutrient elements, as well as dissolvents; and the starchless and leafy vegetables furnish not only the right mineral salts but are the repositories of those elusive but important vitamines, and the "Fat and water solubles," the "A.B.C." foods, whatever those mysterious infinitesimal materials are, while the vegetable fibres furnish a broom to sweep out the intestinal canal.

The nutritive values of the mucusless diet are superior to those of any other foods. This has been demonstrated by results and by the standard tables of food analyses when properly interpreted. Their curative and nutritive values were discovered in this country and Europe at about the same time.

Professor Ehret made the discovery, during his long experience, tests and experiments resulting in his cure, that the grape-sugar of carbohydrates was the source of vitality and vital energy, and not the proteids. This is a fundamental part of the new physiology which he has built up. In 1909 he wrote an article for the European health magazines denouncing the metabolic theory, and in 1912 learned that Thomas Powell, M.D., of Los Angeles had made the same discovery and was effecting wonderful cures by using foods containing what he called "organized carbon," which is the same food ingredient that develops into grape-sugar during digestion.

Man is working against too much friction in his human machine. Hidden away in every part of the human body are thousands of feet of small and almost invisible tubes through which the blood circulates like the water in a water motor. If the blood stream contains sticky mucus from wrong eating, the body machine has to work under continual friction, like a car slowed down by applying the brake. This explains the long-existing mystery of weakness and also that of blood pressure, and the high temperature of fever and inflammation. During the process of healing by the mucusless diet system the same friction occurs, because the mucus is dissolved and is taken into the blood stream. But it occurs periodically, because the blood stream cannot carry it all at once.

The up-to-date fasting and fruit diet have been used dilettantively and without any system and, therefore, failed in most cases. The mucusless diet healing system has been exhaustively tested by the thousands of cures by Professor Ehret and his disciples (the Ehretists) of Europe and the West; especially in advising the procedure in thousands of cases, most of them pronounced "incurable." These have consisted of paralysis, epilepsy, blindness, diabetes, turberculosis, etc.

"The school in which I acquired the knowledge and graduated from," said the originator of the new system, "was in curing my own case of Bright's disease. I am not only fully cured physically but the mental is freed from the depressing and hindering effect of the debris from wrong eating,

and a new life is the result. The only real prevention of disease is found."

During the years, a score of years ago, Ehret in
trying to save his life tried every form of medical
and drugless healing known, mostly with good
reliefs from the latter; but he became discouraged
after each when he discovered that he was not
cured. Not until he combined fasting with fruit and
vegetable diet on his own responsibility was he
healed. In the thousands of cases he has cured since
then he has found the educational factor an important one, that the curing is done by nature's self
healing processes and how they are best assisted.

The healing system must be varied and adapted to
each individual case. The practitioner must have a
practical knowledge of every detail and show in his
own person the results of a perfect cure. The
system combines satisfactorily with any kind of
physical or mental treatments, and gives them
quicker and more satisfactory results.

In one of his books the professor writes of tuberculosis:

"Therewith I also uncover the last secret of consumption. Or does anyone believe that this enormous quantity of mucus thrown off by a patient
stricken with tuberculosis for years and years
emanates from the lung itself? Just because this
patient is then almost forcibly fed on 'mucus' (pap,
milk, fat meats) the mucus can never cease, until
the lung itself decays and the 'bacilli' make their

appearance, when death becomes inevitable. The mystery of the bacilli is solved simply thus: The gradual clogging up of the blood vessels leads to decomposition, to fermentation of these mucus products and 'boiled-dead' food-residues. These decay partially on the living body (pussy abcesses, cancer, tuberculosis, syphillis, lupus, etc.) Now, everybody knows that meat, cheese and all organic matter will again 'germinate, put forth bacilli' during the process of decomposition. It is for this reason that these germs appear and are detectable only in the more advanced stage of the disease, when, however, they are not the cause but the product of the disease, and disease-furthering only in so far as the decomposition, for instance of the lung, is being hastened by them, because of the excretions of the bacilli, their toxins, act poisoning. If it be correct that bacilli invade, 'infect' from the exterior, then it is nothing but the mucus which makes possible their activity, and furnishes the proper soil, the 'disposition'."

Within a period of 14 months Professor Ehret lived 126 days without food, 49 days in one stretch. These fasts (the world-record for absolute scientific observation within an enclosure) were undertaken only after long preparation of the physical organism by a mucusless diet. "I even maintain," said the faster, "that if man lived in accordance with right dietetic laws on a mucusless diet he would experience absolute health, beauty and strength, without pain and grief, just as we are told in the Bible. All so-called miracles by the saints have their origin in ascetics, and are today impossible only

because, although there is much praying done, no
fasting is adhered to. We have no more miracles
because we have no more saints, i.e., sanctified and
healed by ascetics and fastings. The saints were
self-shining, expressed in modern terminology,
medial or radioactive. I wish to state that I myself
have succeeded in visible, electric effluences, but
only by external and internal sun-energies (sun-
baths and food from the 'sun-kitchen,' fruits).

"It is today easier to write books, preach and pray,
saying I am an exception. This is true, but only as
far as pluck and understanding are concerned."

While declaring war on meat and alcohol, Professor
Ehret recognizes that a moderate use of either or
both of these still places one far ahead of the
vegetarian glutton. A person becomes most efficient and develops best in his health if he eats as
little as possible.

A large proportion of ordinary fasting attempts fail
because of the ignorance of the fact that with the
beginning of the mucusless diet the old mucus is
being excreted so much more forcibly until that
person is absolutely clean and healthy. Thus the
seemingly most healthy person has first to pass
through a condition of sickness (cleansing), or go
through an intermediate stage of illness to a higher
level of health.

Growing old is found to be latent disease, a slow
but constantly increasing disturbance in the operation of the motor of life. If, according to Paradisic

primary laws the lungs and skin be given nothing but pure air and sun-electricity, and the stomach and bowels nothing but sun-food (fruits), which are being digested almost without rest, there seems to be no reason why the tube-system of the human body should become defective, weaken, age ,and finally break down entirely. The human organism does not assimilate one atom of mineral substance which has not become organic in the plant. Grape-sugar of the fruits and their nutritive salts, and the salts of the green-leaf starchless vegetables are the right sources for a firm muscle-substance by which a body throws off its diseases and maintains a standard of health. Properly, man in perfect health should exhale fragrance. The stench of sweat, foul breath, etc., indicate but the rotten matter with which nearly all bodies are weighted and handicapped from infancy to that final excess of corruption which stills forever the human engine.

The hairs are odor-tubes or "gas chimneys" and it is no wonder that the pollution they carry off leads to grayness and baldness. The remedy is to be found in the mucusless diet.

Professor Ehret's experimental proof that mucus is the fundamental and main factor in sickness and death differs from the bacillus theory only in the fact that this mucus is the bed, the pre-condition, the primary. The excessive appearance of the white blood corpuscles, i.e., of the white dead mucus, as compared with the red sugar and iron substances is becoming dangerous to life. Red-colored and sweet is the visible token of life and love; white, pale, colorless, bitter, the token of disease and the overwhelming by mucus, the slow dying of the individual. "The death struggle or agony can be regarded only as a last crisis, a final effort of the organism to excrete mucus; a last fight of the still-living cells against the dead ones and their death-poisons."

My first American ancestor, landing in New Amsterdam in 1616, was the colony's first physician, and for three centuries an almost unbroken line of medical men have held up the old tradition. I have been a close student of health and dietetics for a life-time, and it is not lightly that I echo the words of Luther Burbank when the plant wizard paid this tribute, "I have no doubt that Prof. Ehret has found the fundamental cause of all disease." He studied in four continents, keenly alive and observing, familiar with the latest word of science in every phase of his research, yet bringing the genius of the discoverer into play in blazing new paths. Healing himself, experimenting on himself and justifying his conclusions by thousands of cures in his sanitarium and in clinic and by correspondence, he contributed a unique addition to the store of human knowledge. I found him quiet and unassuming, fully alive to the significance of his new teachings but never arrogant nor grasping.

Foreword to the Second Edition

In 1910, part of this book was published as an essay in "Gesundheit" (Health), Zurich, and in the number 17/18 edition of "Lebenskunst" (Art of Life), publisher K. Lentze, Leipzig. It aroused such great interest and demand that I felt obliged to publish it in book form with considerably more detail and important additions in the text.

Within one year the first 5,000 copies of "Rational Fasting" were sold out, which is proof enough of its great popularity. And I hope that this second edition will find an even larger audience who will listen to the truth it contains. Apart from a few minor additions, the content of my book was not altered.

May this book serve all readers seeking after truth regardless of its source; may it especially serve the sick and encourage those worrying about the loss of their youth and the first signs of old age.

Locarno, Autumn 1912

ARNOLD EHRET.

Foreword to the Third Edition

There has been such great demand and praise for "Rational Fasting" that a third edition has become necessary. In the meantime, nature doctors have also released publications on fasting cures despite their initial objection to the most natural of all cures. However, they obviously still lack the understanding that there is only ONE disease, i.e. all diseases are related in that they have a common fundamental cause. Therefore, fasting and keeping to a natural diet will help in all cases of sickness, however, it will not help all patients without exception.

Even in the United States my book has become a bestseller as is apparent from a letter I received from Dr. Benedict Lust, owner and director of the first natural health spa in the United States (New Jersey). Dr. Lust, who is also the editor of "Nature's Path" magazine, writes on July 23rd as follows:

"The book market here is absolutely saturated with publications on fasting. Dewey, Haskell, Sinclair, etc. to name but a few authors. However, no one has so deeply and accurately grasped the problem than you in your book which we welcome

with great delight. It certainly is the best both
from a practical and scientifically sound point of
view. I really wished I had the financial means to
publish your book and distribute it by the mil-
lions."

There is a disconcerting indication that fasting will
become nothing but a fad. Hopefully, my cure will
be spared that fate and gradually establish itself in
a permanent first place to the benefit of all people.

Locarno, Summer 1914.

                              ARNOLD EHRET.

Preface

Today's thinking indicates one fundamental difference to former times namely that everybody has a different concept about the reason for being. Not even the scientists who are specializing in Natural Sciences are in accord among themselves. They are asking more and more questions, make everything more questionable and finally make man a living question mark.

Mauthner in his criticisms on linguistics reveals a secret everybody already knows: "nowadays all questions are answered with an equal amount of 'yes' and 'no'. Everything that has been proven has also been disproven. The most controversial among all differing opinions and scientific controversies is that of the meaning of disease.

I feel I should not wait any longer with making my experience public; however my message is not intended for just everybody, it is dedicated to those who are in search of truth and can recognize and accept facts on the strength of actual experiments without bothering to question who proclaimed them and whether the majority agrees with them or disagrees with them.

A year ago the magazine "Vegetarian Watch Tower" published a report how my first disciple and myself purposely went to the malaria infested provinces of Italy in order to test our resistance to this fever at a pulse beat of 45/52. We made it a point to sleep outdoors in areas that were considered highly contagious, and indulged in strenuous endurance marches during the day. I have offered my services to all European and American authorities to use my experience in order to make people positively fever resistant. I still maintain today that I am immune to cholera—and I am ready to prove it—and would not contract it even if I were to eat non-ripened fruit. More than that, I maintain that I could help make other people resistant if they were to live according to my advice. It is my duty and moral obligation to perpetuate the truth which I have experienced on my own body and which will serve the healthy to remain strong and not to fall prey to disease and sickness.

Nowadays there are two ways for sick people to combat their illness. There is the one kind of sick who want to get it over and done with as soon as possible. They take pills, drugs, vaccines etc. and indeed these medications will help to restore their health for a while. However a complete cure becomes less likely in the long run and eventually a renewed and more severe breakdown of the system is unavoidable.

Man seems to think this is the way it should be and medical science therefore complies superbly with the demands made upon it for instant cure. There is no denying the medical accomplishments.

The other kind of patient oftentimes considered somewhat old fashioned but in effect the one that is honest with himself, intelligent and concerned about the origin of the illness that has befallen him, wants to get at the heart of things and cure himself once and for all. To achieve this end there will have to be sacrifices. The patient becomes his own doctor and adviser. All I can do is show him the way. This is the purpose of this book.

Naturopathy works within these two extremes. Whilst cautioning against overindulgence in foods —the main cause for most diseases—and prevention are given only somewhat secondary importance, Naturopathy does contribute greatly by applying natural ways of healing and it cannot be denied that by her methods including the use of fresh air and water treatments, the success of the fasting cure would be even further increased.

This booklet will give a general outline what a fast should be like and which foods are to be avoided but it must be remembered that the individual's personal requirements may vary from one case to the next and proper advice should always be sought. I am confident that my readers who have already gained good insight into my theory will profit even more from this extensive writing.

It appears that the medical association has tradi-

tionally very little use for the discoveries of a
non-professional but that just can't be helped.
Science and particularly natural science and tech-
nology have never questioned the qualifications of
the great discoverers. The world might have made
fun occasionally of amateurs like Franklin and
Galvani, Edison and Zeppelin but their genius was
nevertheless recognized and respected. The medical
school however may teach about the Priessnitz
compress and never mention at all that he too was
a non-professional.

I do not share the animosity of the Naturopaths
toward the medical profession nor do I sanction,
indeed I condemn, the activities of any quack who
is carrying on his activities under the pretext of
'nature cures'.—

These are a few of my thoughts.

CHAPTER 1

The common fundamental cause in the nature of diseases

From the earliest periods of civilization onward and throughout all phases in the development of medical science it was commonly believed that diseases were of external nature. By entering into the human body they disrupted its normal functions, caused pain and eventually destroyed it completely. Even modern medical science, no matter how enlightened it pretends to be, has not quite abandoned this basic belief. Indeed, bacteriologists rejoice over every newly discovered bacillus as further indication of the external danger to man's health.

Looking at it from a philosophical point of view we find that a change in its name is the only difference between the mediaeval conception of the so called 'evil spirit' on the one hand and the proven existence of the microscopically visible 'bacillus' of modern times on the other.

There is, however, still the question of man's varying degree of susceptibility which nobody so far has explained to us. Tests indicate of course symptoms and reactions thereto but they really do not prove anything because the bacteria were

injected directly into the blood-stream instead of
entering orally and then proceeding into the digestive channel. There is something to the concept of
an invasion of a disease—even a hereditary one—
into the body from without, however not in the
sense that the invader is an evil spirit hostile to life,
or a microscopic bacillus; rather, all diseases without exception including the hereditary ones are
caused—not counting a few which are due to
insufficient hygiene—by biologically wrong, unnatural foods and by each ounce of over-eating.

First of all I maintain that during all diseases
without exception the organism tends to secrete a
kind of mucus, and in case of a more advanced
stage it takes the form of pus (decomposed blood).
[It is understood that every healthy organism
contains a certain amount of fatty substances.]
Every professional will agree to this whether we
speak of catarrhal diseases ranging from nasal drip
to chest cold, to inflammation of the lungs and to
consumption. Even when the secretion of mucus is
not visible to the eye as in cases of ear, eye, skin or
stomach trouble, heart diseases, rheumatism, gout,
etc., even in all degrees of insanity, mucus is still
the main cause of the illness. When the natural
secretive organs become unable to cope with the
disposal of the excess mucus, it will enter into the
blood stream and cause heat, inflammation, pain
and fever at such spots where the vessel system has
contracted which could be due to a cold.

We need only to give any patient nothing but
'mucusless' food, for instance fruit or even nothing

but water or lemonade; and we would find that the now made idle entire digestive energy would attack the mucus matter accumulated since childhood and frequently hardened, as well as the so called 'pathological beds' (decomposed cellular tissues). And the result? With absolute certainty this mucus which I consider as the common main cause of all diseases will appear in the urine and in the excrements. If the disease is somewhat more advanced and the patient has developed deposits of decomposed cellular tissues, then pus is also being secreted. Once the formation of mucus by means of 'artifical' food, fatty meats, bread, potatoes, farinaceous products, rice, milk, etc., ceases, the blood itself attacks the mucus and the pus in the body and secretes them through the urine, and in the case of heavily infected bodies even through all the openings at its command as for instance also through the mucus membranes.

If potatoes, grain meal, rice or meat are boiled long enough, we get jelly-like slime (mucus) or paste similar to the kind that is used by bookbinders and carpenters. This slimy substance soon turns sour, ferments, and forms a bed for fungi, molds and bacilli. During digestion, which is nothing else but a boiling, a combustion, this slime or paste is created in the same manner, for the blood can use only the converted dextrose sugar transformed from starch. The waste matter, this superfluous product, i.e., this paste or slime is at first completely excreted. It is however easy to understand that in the course of one's lifetime the intestines and the stomach are gradually pasted and slimed up to such an extent that this paste or flora and this slime of fauna origin turn into fermentation, clog up the blood vessels and finally decompose the stagnated blood.

If figs, dates or grapes are boiled into a pap we get a kind of thick syrup which however does not ferment and never leaves slime. It is true that fruit sugar, the most important thing for the blood, is also sticky, but it is completely absorbed by the body since it represents the highest form of combustible substance and leaves for excretion only traces of cellulose which not being sticky are promptly disposed of and do not ferment. Owing to its resistance to fermentation, boiled down sugar is even used for the preservation of various foods.

Each healthy or sick person develops a sticky mucus on the tongue as soon as he cuts down on his intake of food or goes on a fast. This occurs also on the mucus membrane of the stomach of which the tongue is an exact copy. In the first stool after a fast this mucus makes its appearance. I recommend to you and physicians and researchers to test my claims by way of experiments which alone are entitled to real scientific recognition. The experiment, the question put to nature, is the basis of all natural science and reveals the infallible truth, no matter whether it is stated by me or somebody else. Furthermore, I recommend the following experiments to those who are brave enough to test on their own bodies what I undertook on mine. They will receive the same answer from nature, i.e., from their organism, provided that the latter is 'healthy' in my interpretation of the word. Only the cleansed, healthy mucusless organism reacts with a certain predictable exactness. After a two year strict fruit diet with interspersed fasting cures, I had attained a degree of health which is simply not imaginable nowadays and which allowed me to make the following experiments:

I made an incision in my lower arm with a knife: there was no flow of blood because it thickened instantly closing up the wound, no inflammation, no pain, no mucus and pus, healed up in three days, blood crust thrown off. Later, with vegetarian food, including mucus forming starch food, but without eggs and milk, the wound bled a little, caused some pain and pussed slightly, a light inflammation, and complete healing only after some time. After a meat diet and some alcohol the same type of wound bled longer, the blood of a light color, red and thin, inflammation, pain, pussing for several days, and healing only after a two-day fast.

I have offered myself in vain to the Prussian Ministry of War for a repetition of this experiment. Why is it that the wounds of the Japanese healed much faster and better in the Russo-Japanese war than those of the 'meat and brandy Russians'? Has nobody, for 2,000 years, ever wondered why the opening of the artery and even the poison cup could not kill Seneca who had despised meat and fasted in prison? It is said that even before he was imprisoned Seneca took nothing but fruit and water.

In the final analysis all disease is nothing more than a clogging up of the smallest blood vessels, the capillaries, with mucus. Nobody would want to clean out the water pipe system of a city into which the pumps had fed dirty water which in turn clogged up the filters, without having the water supply shut off during the cleaning process. If the conduit supplies the entire city or a portion of it with unclean water or even if only some of the smaller pipes were clogged up, nobody in the world would think of just repairing the defective spot; everybody thinks at once to go to the main feed and the filters, and these together with the pumps can be cleaned only as long as the water supply is shut off.

If I were to paraphrase the First Commandment, this is what it would be: "I am the Lord, thy physician". Nature alone heals, cleanses and eliminates mucus without fail, but only if the intake of at least the mucus producing foods is stopped. Each physiological system—that of man and animal alike—cleanses itself automatically and with tireless effort dissolves the mucus in the clogged up vessels as soon as at least the supply of solid food has been interrupted. Even in the case of the supposedly healthy man, this mucus, as already mentioned, will then appear in the urine where it can be seen after cooling off in the proper glass tubes! Whoever denies, ignores or rejects this fundamental fact perhaps because it goes against his grain or is not scientific enough for him, joins those who are guilty of obstructing the path to the discovery of the principal causes for all diseases. This is of course in the first place to his own detriment.

This will also unveil the ultimate secret of consumption. Or does anybody believe that the enormous amount of mucus coughed up by a tuberculosis patient year after year emanates only from the lungs themselves? Since such patients are many times nourished with high mucus producing foods such as pap, milk and fatty meats, the lungs remain under constant strain and finally disintegrate and thereby provide the perfect breeding grounds for the bacilli which will launch the deathly final attack. The mystery of the bacilli is thus simply solved: the gradual clogging up of the blood vessels with mucus leads to decomposition and fermentation of these mucus food residues. They decay partially in the living body (pussy abcesses, cancer, tuberculosis, syphilis, lupus, etc.). Now everybody knows that meat, cheese and all organic matter will again 'germinate, put forth bacilli' during the process of decomposition. It is for this reason that these new germs appear and are detectable only in the more advanced stage of the disease. They are not the cause but the end product of the disease and speed up the process of decomposition of the lung for example through excretions of poisonous toxins. If it were true that bacilli invade from the exterior, then it is nothing but the mucus which permits them their activity and furnishes the proper predisposition.

As mentioned before I have repeatedly (at one time for as long as two years) lived on a mucusless diet, i.e., on fruit exclusively. As a result I could do without a handkerchief which product of civilization I hardly need even up to this date. Has anyone ever seen a wild healthy animal spit or blow its nose?

I was suffering from a chronic inflammation of the kidneys considered incurable. But, not only was I cured, I am also enjoying a degree of health and efficiency which far surpasses even that of my healthiest youth. Show me the man who having been near death at 31, eight years later can run continuously for two and a quarter hours or take an endurance hike lasting 56 hours!

Surely it is theoretically correct that man was a mere fruit eater in times gone by, and biologically correct, that he can be it even today. There is no proof necessary of the fact since plain common sense will tell that man lived on fruits only before he became a hunter. I even maintain that he lived in absolute health, beauty and strength without pain and grief just the way the Bible says.—Fruit alone, the sole mucusless food, is natural. Everything prepared by man, or supposedly improved by him, is evil. The evidence regarding fruit is scientifically proven; the apple or banana for instance contain everything that man needs. Man is so perfect that he can live on only one kind of fruit for at least quite some time. But nature's self-evident truth must not be ignored just because nobody has been able to apply it in practice on account of the inhibitions which civilization has imposed on us. From eating only fruit one brings about a crisis, i.e., cleansing. No man would have ever believed me that it was possible to live without food for 126 days during 14 months in which 49 days were undertaken at a stretch. Now that I have done it, this truth is still not understood. Up to now I have stated and taught only that fruit is the most natural remedy. However, the self-evident is not always easily believed. When in the previous century somebody talked about telephoning from London to Paris, everybody laughed because there had never been such a thing. Natural foods are not very popular any more because almost no one eats them and man being a product of civilization cannot easily come by them. It must also be remembered that there are other interest groups which fear that the prices of artificial foodstuffs may drop, and still others that fear physicians might become unnecessary. The latter need not worry for any fasting and fruit cure requires very strict observation and instruction. Therefore more doctors are needed for fewer patients who, however, will gladly pay more if they get well. Thus, the concern regarding the doctors' existence is unfounded.

Almost all attempts at fasting fail on account of the ignorance of the faster as to all that is involved. One fact must be carefully borne in mind, namely that at the beginning of the mucusless diet there will be the startling discovery that a lot of the old mucus is being excreted and quite forcibly so until that person is absolutely clean and healthy. THUS

THE SEEMINGLY HEALTHY PERSON HAS FIRST TO PASS THROUGH A CONDITION OF SICKNESS (CLEANSING), or go through an intermediate stage of illness in order to attain a higher level of health. This is the big hurdle which even many vegetarians have failed to take and consequently rejected the credibility of this highest truth just like the mass of people are doing. I have contributed my experience to the "Vegetarian Watch-Tower" and substantiated my method by stating my experiments and the facts I had gathered during my 49 day fast and the preceding fruit diet. This served to refute the greatest objection, the fear of undernourishment. My state of health was only improved by this radical excretion of mucus, not counting a few unhygienic circumstances during the test. I received numerous letters of appreciation especially from the educated classes. Most vegetarians however unheedingly mucus ahead. The foods which they brand as poisonous: meat, alcohol, coffee and tobacco are by comparison rather harmless in the long run AS LONG AS THEY ARE CONSUMED WITH MODERATION.

In order to avoid misunderstanding on the part of teetotalers and vegetarians, I must insert a few explanations here. Meat is not a food, it is only a stimulant which ferments and decays in the stomach. The process of decay, however, does not begin in the stomach, it sets in right after the slaughtering of the animal. Such are Prof. Dr. S. Graham's findings after various experiments and I enlarge even further in this respect: meats act as stimulants through the very poisons due to decay which lead to the mistaken notion that it is a strengthening food. Or is there anyone who contends that the albumen molecule after having gone through the process of decay will regenerate itself in the stomach and subsequently celebrate its resurrection in some muscle of the human body? Of course not! Like alcohol, at first meat simulates a feeling of strength and energy until the entire organism is clogged up by it and the breakdown becomes inevitable. All other stimulants act likewise.

The basic evil of all non-vegetarian forms of diet lies always in the overeating of meat which in turn brings on other evils, notably the craving for alcohol. Man who nourishes himself on fruit will soon lose his desire for alcoholic beverages whereas the meat eater is constantly tempted by it since meat produces thirst. Alcohol acts as a kind of antidote to meat and the big city gourmand who eats mostly meats must therefore indulge himself in wines, coffee and smoking in order to at least in some way counteract meat poisoning. It is a well known fact that one feels decidedly fresher, physically and mentally, after a moderate dinner even if made up of such foods as are considered 'stimulants' as compared to stuffing oneself to the brim with the so-called good foods from the vegetarian kitchen.

I ABSOLUTELY DECLARE WAR ON MEAT AND ALCOHOL. But whoever finds it impossible to give up meat and alcohol entirely is still far

ahead of the vegetarian glutton provided he eats
moderately. The American, Fletcher proved with
tremendous success that a person becomes most
efficient and healthiest if he eats as little as
possible. This is the secret I discovered also on the
basis of my own experiments. Are not the poorer
people who by necessity must eat more moderately
throughout the years, also the ones that become
oldest? Have not the greatest discoverers and in-
ventors sprung from the less privileged classes, i.e.,
been small eaters? And were not the greatest of
mankind, the prophets, founders of religions, etc.,
ascetics? What culture is this, to wine and dine
three times a day; or do we understand by social
progress that each working man must eat five times
a day and then drink a lot of beer at night? Since
the sick organism can regenerate itself without
being given food, then it follows that a healthy
organism needs but little food in order to retain its
health, strength and perseverance.

All miracles performed by saints at the so-called
holy places have become rare for the simple reason
that, although much praying is done, not much
fasting is adhered to. We don't have miracles any
more because we have no more saints, no more
blessed and healed by asceticism and fasting. The
saints were radiant not by special grace but
through divine healthy asceticism. I just wish to
mention here that I myself have succeeded in
visible electric effluences, but only by external and
internal sun energies (sun baths and food from the
sun kitchen: fruit).

The entire world is mystified by the miracles of ancient times. And yet, the answers can be found in simple experiments which everybody can repeat if he is brave enough. But it is apparently easier to write books, preach and pray, or to say that I am an exception. This is true but only so far as courage and knowledge are concerned. Physiologically all men are equal. If man eats moderately and is healthy, he will also be able to indulge himself at times in meats and starches without any problem of digestion and elimination of mucus residues thus produced. He would of course further improve his health if he ate only fruit of which he needs but little because it is the most perfect nourishment there is. Nature is difficult for man to accept because he has built himself up of overcooked food and his cells are condemned to death. Every time he exposes himself to the sun or eats the living cells of fruit, or engages in a fast all this dead matter is eliminated from his body. However, the cure of fasting must be carried out with the greatest care.

Today's medications are designed to protect man from a breakdown of his cells but in most cases a doctor will only be consulted when the disease is imminent whereas very little if anything is done for prevention.

The vegetarians cannot deny that the meat and alcohol consuming portion of the population has produced a good number of healthy people, capable of great achievements and longevity. At a closer look however, it will turn out that such individuals usually belong to the group of moderate eaters. Overeating is less harmful in the case of meat eaters because meat contains proportionally less mucus than starches of which vegetarian food is oftentimes made up not to mention the celebrated vegetarian dinners with entirely too many dishes. I myself have not bothered much about meals for many years now; I eat only when I have appetite and then so little that it does not cause any harmful effect if and when on occasion I am obliged to eat something which is not free from objection.

If the most serious diseases can be cured by fasting which has been proven thousands of times and if one gets even stronger during the fast—provided it is applied correctly—it then stands to reason that a diet of fruit should have an even more positive effect. This point has been scientifically proven by the highly regarded Dr. Bircher. It is true that the science of natural healing has recognized the fact that the sick organism has to get 'rid of something' in order to get better. Therefore it was considered of greatest importance to eliminate meat and alcohol from the patients diet but only very little attention was paid to the most effective element in the healing process: abstinence, restraint and the fruit diet. This does not mean much in the face of my 'mucus theory'. It is unbelievable how much evil has been attributed to the 'mucusless' alcohol. Soon enough it will be made the scapegoat of all diseases simply because a few unfortunate alcoholics ended in delirium. I maintain that if an alcoholic were to be made to fast for a few days or eat nothing but fruit, he would soon lose his taste for beer and wine. This proves that the entire civilized mass of foods from beefsteak to seemingly harmless oatmeals creates a desire for these detestable antidotes: alcohol, coffee, tea, tobacco. Why? Because overeating makes man lazy and consequently he has to pep himself up with stimulants. The true reason then for an increase in the alcohol consumption is overeating, especially with meat. Dr. Graham says in his "Physiology of Nourishment": "A drinker can reach a high age, a glutton never." This is correct because alcohol acts as a stimulant, especially beer and is less harmful in the long run than the chronically clogged up digestive channel with mucus food.

Now let me ask what sounds more reasonable to you: to subjugate the body to all kinds of medication, injections, vaccinations and possibly even operations, or to try to rid the body of the poisonous mucus accumulated since childhood in the cellular tissues, by reducing the intake of food?

Not even the best chef could produce something more perfect and more mucusless than an apple, a grape or banana. If over-eating and the consumption of high mucus producing foods is the true fundamental cause of all diseases without exception—and I maintain that everybody could obtain the proof to this effect from his own body—then there exists but one natural remedy: fasting and fruit diet.

It is a well known fact that animals take to fasting at the slightest feeling of being unwell. Even our domestic animals whose sharp instincts for the right kind of nourishment have otherwise been greatly reduced by their environment and the food man has been feeding them, will nevertheless when sick accept only the most essential foods and take to fasting until they are better. By contrast man is not permitted such natural ways of healing himself. Under no circumstances must he live on short rations for more than one or two days for fear that he may lose strength.

Many physicians have recognized the merits of fasting, some speak of miraculous cures, others of cure for the uncurable, cure of all cures, etc. Unfortunately there are always some quacks around who have nothing better to do than to misrepresent and thereby discredit a good thing. This is particularly deplorable in the case of my fasting cure which requires extreme care in its execution. I have accomplished most significant results through my world record breaking 49 day fast (see "The Vegetarian Watch-Tower" 1909, book 19, 20, 22, 1920 book 1 and 2). Furthermore I am the only one who combines this cure with a systematically and individually adapted fruit diet, which makes the fast astonishingly easier to carry through and absolutely harmless. We are, therefore in a position to heal diseases which the school of medicine designates as incurable. In view of my conclusions that the mucus residues are the fundamental cause and main factor in the nature of all diseases, symptoms of old age, obesity, baldness, wrinkles, nervous disorders and loss of memory, etc., there is justified hope for a new phase in the development of more progressive healing methods and biological medicine.

Hippocrates recognized the uniformity in the formation of diseases. Prof. Jaeger has defined this common cause as a kind of stench but he didn't discover the source of this 'bad smell'. Dr. Lahmann and some of his colleagues, especially Kuhne, directed their research to the common cause of foreign matter. But not one of them recognized the fact that it is the mucus produced by the unnatural foods which clogs up our organisms from childhood on, tends to ferment, forms pathological beds, and in the end decomposes the cellular tissues of the body. During colds or high temperature the mucus gets occasionally loosened up, and in its endeavour to leave the body it creates all sorts of disturbing symptoms. These have oftentimes been regarded as the disease itself. It is therefore possible for the first time to define the various degrees of susceptibility to disease. The more mucus being administered to the body from childhood on, and the less mucus being excreted— in some cases this is due to hereditary weakness in the organs which are to perform this task—the greater is man's susceptibility to catch cold, fever, to freeze, to invite bacilli, to get sick and to grow old. Very likely this discovery will contribute to lift the veil that has hitherto always surrounded the nature of the white blood corpuscles. I believe that we are dealing here with one of the errors of medical science. Contrary to common belief I maintain that the bacteria, when they enter the body, attack the white blood corpuscles and not

the other way round, for the white corpuscles
consist to a large extent of just that famous mucus
described in such detail during the preceding pages.
Bacteria are being bred outside of the organism on
mucus rich potatoes, broth, gelatine, etc. Mucus is
a nitrogenous, vegetable or animal substance consisting of an alkaline reacting fluid which contains
granulated cells of the same appearance as the
white blood corpuscles. Perhaps in an entirely
healthy body the so-called mucus membrane
should not be all white and slimy but clean and red
like that in animals. Mucus might even be a chief
contributor to wide-spread paleness.

By means of this 'mucus theory' we have come to
explain away much of the mystery of disease. He
who believes in the conclusions derived from my
experiments benefits in three important ways: he
can heal himself not only where all else has failed,
he can learn to make himself strong and condition
himself to be less if at all susceptible to disease.

The human organism is mechanically speaking a
complicated system of tubes and blood vessels
which is given its impetus through the air in the
lungs. The blood fluid in turn is constantly kept
moving and regulated by the heart as the main
valve. The air which we breathe in is separated in
the lungs into oxygen and nitrogen, thus the blood
is constantly kept moving and the human body
functions for a long time without getting tired.
Therefore the matter is simple: If the mechanism is
not overburdened with too much food, it will
perform at its best and not slow down. I cannot

accept the usual argument that nature absolutely demands that man must indulge in lots of 'good eating' so that he can perform his daily tasks. Such people have to first find out for themselves for how long it is possible to work or walk without fatigue after a fast or a fruit diet.

In the first place fatigue means a reduction in strength by too much digestive activity, secondly a clogging up of the blood vessels and thirdly a certain internal poisoning due to excretion of excess mucus. All organic substances of animal origin excrete poisonous cyan groups in their decomposition, which the chemist Hensel has defined as bacilli proper. The air is not only the most important and most perfect manipulator of the human body but it is also most essential to build strength and reserves. Very likely the animal organism obtains nitrogen also from the air. It has been stated that certain caterpillars increased their weight through intake of air alone.

CHAPTER 2

Remedies for the removal of the common fundamental cause and the prevention of their recurrence

Having told my readers about the horrors of being sick or falling sick, it befits me now to give a summary—as far as this can be expressed in general terms—of how to deal successfully with mucus poisoning, this greatest foe of health, by fasting and keeping a proper diet.

Healthy people can submit to a fasting cure without any further ceremony. It goes without saying that they must fast reasonably, i.e. avoid dangerous overexertions during the fasting period by not demanding of themselves physical or mental performances which they could not live up to even at full fare. Also, a precautionary measure must be taken at the beginning of the fast: the complete emptying of the bowels. A harmless purgative (such as a mild herbal laxative), a syringe, or both should be used. The reasoning behind this is that he who fasts should not be bothered unnecessarily by gas or decomposing matter which form from the excrements remaining in the bowels. It suffices, as already stated, that the mucus during the excretion will give him enough trouble.

If the reader, although healthy, does not dare take

a more prolonged fast, he should try a short one. A thirty-six hour fast, once or twice a week, will in time produce very favorable results. It is best to start such a fast by skipping supper, taking an enema instead. Then, abstain from food until the morning following the full day of fasting. Breakfast that morning should consist of nothing but fruit. Eating fruit is necessary after each fasting, as the fruit juices cause the now loosened mucus to move. Let me caution, in the case of sick and old people this treatment must be carefully individualized.

A longer fast, say for 3 days, done in the way described above and followed by what I call an after-fasting cure, will naturally show results much quicker. That is, do not eat anything for three days and drink only fresh lemonade, unsugared, in single gulps as may become necessary. On the fourth day eat some fruit and take a thorough enema in the evening. Then add more fruit from day to day, so that by about the seventh day of the after-cure the normal quantity of fruit-diet in the proper composition and selection has been reached.

Healthy persons, especially those whose occupation permits them to spend some time in bed in case of difficult excretions of mucus, can extend the fasting cure for weeks. Nobody should seriously object to the so-called "bad looks" or the decrease in weight during this period; the body "fasts itself into health", despite the miserable complexion. Within a remarkably short time the cheeks will be adorned by a healthy, natural red and the weight restored to its normal standard, since after a fast the body reacts to every ounce of food. Incidentally, moderate eaters and frequently fasting people have a very fine, spiritual facial expression, for instance, it is said that Pope Leo XIII, that great faster, had a very clear, almost transparent complexion.

The success of any fasting cure depends also to a great extent on the attitude of the person submitting to it. By no means should he permit himself to become depressed or ill-humored. During the disagreeable moments, some may prefer to rest, others may decide to do some light and mechanical work.

When the body has been rid of the mucus, slime and paste, then it is the sacred duty of the person who has regained health to keep up the reclaimed highest earthly happiness and to guard it by means of natural, correct food. On this subject a few short remarks in the following paragraphs will not come amiss.

Persons with acute health problems, lung or heart trouble for instance, may not be able to fast, however, they can stop further accumulation of mucus by adhering to a proper diet. All mucus formers, especially flour (pastries), rice, potatoes, boiled milk, cheese, meat, etc. should be avoided. Whoever cannot do without bread entirely, should eat brown or white bread only, toasted. By toasting the bread, it loses much of its harmfulness, as the mucus substances are partly destroyed. Furthermore, toast has the added advantage that it cannot be gulped down and the necessary chewing

will fatigue us, so that we eat less. If, on account of
bad teeth, eating toasted bread poses a problem,
suck on it until it dissolves. As to potatoes, if at all,
eat them only baked and be sure and eat the
jackets.

At this point, many a reader will probably question
what, if any, "nutritious food" remains. Unfortunately, it is not possible for me to go into the
question of food and its effects exhaustively in this
book and a few statements have to suffice. As to
the value of meat, it is a known fact that the body
requires only a slight amount of albumin contained
in the meat. Sugary fruits will fully cover this
demand. Bananas and nuts combined with a few
figs or dates, for instance, are first class muscle
formers and provide the body with energy. In fact,
green salads, prepared with oil and plenty of
lemon, and all the delicious fruits and berries,
including those from the South, are excellent
nutritious food. And when springtime comes, and
least season's fruits, especially apples, are on the
decline, and the new vegetables not yet ready, does
not Mother Nature help us out abundantly with
oranges from the South? Will the aroma and wealth
of these splendid products of nature not induce
man to eventually become a fruit-eater entirely?
More detail on fasting and a balanced fruit-diet is
set forth in my "Mucusless Diet Healing System".

It may be well to mention also that non-fasters and
people suffering from a slight ailment should at
least follow the morning fast or non-breakfast plan.
It would, indeed, be better for everybody not to

eat anything before 10 o'clock and then nothing but fruit. The reward for this little chastising will certainly show itself, if kept up faithfully.

Now, just one more word to those who think it impossible to give up the usual mucus food (meat, etc.). To those "unfortunate ones" I give this advice: Chew your food, that is every bite, thoroughly as recommended by the American, Fletcher, in one word "fletcherize." Not that the fruit-eaters should not do this, certainly, but the poison-laden mucus eaters must do so especially, if they do not wish to sink into their graves all too soon. Chewing slowly furthers the secretion of saliva which decreases the formation of mucus and prevents overeating. Of course, this class of people cannot quite achieve the standard of health and strength, preservation of youth and perseverance, physical and mental capacity of the faster and fruit-eater.

Once man is healthy in my sense of the word by fasting and following a fruit-diet, that is, free from mucus, slime and germ, he, if he stays with the fruit-diet, need not fast any longer. And only then will he find a pleasure in eating which he never dreamt of before. Only in this way will man find the way to happiness, harmony and the solution of all questions, as only through this he can become want-free and get "nearest to divinity."

The fundamental cause of growing old and ugly

Nature's Ways to Maintain Youth and Beauty

I will now follow up the previous general remarks to the effect that mucus is the main cause of disease and the aging process with particular reference to its influence over the development of all the vital organs. I will show how it impairs beauty and instead produces symptoms of ugliness and age.

If we could have the perfect Paradisaic situation where the lungs and skin would take in nothing but pure air and sun, and the stomach and bowels be fed nothing but natural foods, i.e. fruits, which are digested almost without leaving any residues, then only mucusless, pasteless and germless cellulose would be secreted from the body and there seems to be no reason why the vessel system should become defective, weaken, age and finally break down entirely. The living energy cells of fruit which should constitute the best part of our diet are often neglected in favor of meat products etc. which in their raw condition are meant for beasts of prey, but are chemically changed by air-oxidation (decay), overcooked and thus robbed of their energy by the time we consume them. Mucus accumulates especially in the stomach and bowels and slowly clogs up the whole organism including the glands. In the final analysis this causes chronic defects, helps the aging process and is the main factor in the nature of all disease. Growing old, therefore, is a latent disease, that is, a slow but constant increase in the slowdown of the motor of life.

The study of the chemical composition of our food products indicates that there is a decided lack of minerals in boiled food.

The question arises whether faded beauty, human ugliness and symptoms of growing old can be traced back to nourishment. If this were so, then beauty treatments and rejuvenation would require a dietetic therapy and an improvement in our eating habits. But inasmuch as beauty, especially human beauty, cannot be defined in absolute terms since everybody has a different taste, I will limit myself to more or less the standard demands made of aesthetic beauty. The sickly paleness of modern man can hardly be termed as beautiful. It is the result of the wrong foods we eat. What a wonderfully healthy color we could have if our diet consisted of grapes, cherries and oranges, etc. and our hobbies of outdoor activities. The presence of mucus indicates the absence of enough mineral substances which in turn are responsible for this lack of color. Just compare the food tables of Dr. Konig and you will find that the mucusless food, fruit and vegetables, rank highest as regards their mineral content, especially lime. The size of a person, i.e., his frame and bone structure depends for instance mainly on the amount of lime contained in the food. The Japanese want to increase the size of their race by eating more meat. They are certainly ill advised. All reduction in size, deformities, and especially tooth decay are due to lack of lime. Modern cooking boils the lime right out of milk and vegetables. The tremendous lack of minerals in today's food, especially in meat as compared with fruit, will be made responsible for the emergence of a toothless human race. This may sound like a figment of the imagination but it is quite a serious thought in which many doctors have joined. Where fruit would be the answer to the existing deficiency, inorganic substances have been chosen as substitute. The human organism does not assimilate one single atom of mineral substance which has not become organic. We have lived with one of the evils of civilization—obesity— for so long that our aesthetic feeling in this regard has become somewhat disturbed and we do not even know what constitutes normal any longer. I personally do not consider the overly developed muscular man particularly beautiful and a standard of the ideal. Weight, shape and especially the frame of the body are too big. Every accumulation of fat is pathological and in this sense not aesthetic. No animal living in freedom grows fat like modern man. The reason is simply too much food and too much to drink resulting in sluggishness and clogging up of the bodily organism. The dextrose sugar and all other nutritive attributes of fruit are the real muscle builders and regenerators of the demoralized body.

Facial and bodily flabbiness have become quite commonplace. It is ugly and certainly pathological. Curiously enough this flabbiness is considered

beautiful, and more than that, it is admired as an
indication of abundant health, while our experience teaches us quite to the contrary that the slim,
youthful person has more strength and per-
severence and generally reaches greater longevity.

Rarely if ever will you see an obese 80 or 90 year
old. The ultimate irony is that there exists a
tendency to believe that tuberculosis can be "fat-
tened' away. If fat people do not die in their best
years of a stroke or a heart attack, their bodies
become sluggish and their desire for food decreases
in spite of all artificial stimulations of the appetite.
The skin, especially of the face, having been under
extreme tension for years folds and wrinkles. It has
lost its youthful elasticity on account of insufficient and unhealthy blood circulation as well as
lack of light and sun. No facial massage or beauty
treatment will do much good at this late stage. The
distinction and beauty of the facial features, the
purity and healthy color of the complexion, the
clarity and natural size of the eyes, the charm of
expression and the color of the lips, they all age
and turn ugly as an outward indication of what is
going on inside the clogged up organism. We have
concluded previously that the stomach and the
bowels are the main deposit centers of our famous
mucus from which most symptoms of diseases
emanate, including the process of aging.

What is sometimes talked about as 'the beautiful
roundness of the cheeks' is quite deceiving. More
often than not it is accompanied by a swelling of
the nose, a good indication of the presence of
mucus matter.

The preservation of the hair

Reasons for becoming bald and gray

I will now discuss the most important and most striking symptom of growing old: getting gray hair and getting bald. An entire section must be devoted to this problem because its occurrence generally causes great concern and is considered one of the first indications of getting old to which even science has hitherto not had any comforting answer.

The fashion for males and females has been to wear their hair extremely short for quite a few years now so that we have become accustomed to this look as well as that of the frightening proportion of bald heads among us. This voluntary and involuntary absence of hair has caused us to lose our artistic sense for the aesthetic pleasures which the harmonic creation of man once inspired in us. Man who is not only intellectually but also aesthetically speaking, the crowning glory of creation has been robbed of the splendid crown on his head, his hair. They could be called 'walking skulls' these beardless, colorless and expressionless heads of today. Just imagine the most beautiful woman without hair! Which man wouldn't turn away with horror?

On the other hand I cannot blame anybody for preferring the clean shaven look to the positively unaesthetic appearance of some of the people who do wear long hair and beards. In our time of conformity it is preferred, and rightfully so, to cut off this odorous, ugly, disheveled, uneven and hereditarily morbid hair which would otherwise be quite a good indication of the condition of man's organism. It stands to reason to surmise that any outward manifestation of physical degeneration reflects internal disturbances of the organism. Nature reveals such disturbances oftentimes through disharmony of shape and color. Doubters of my point of view and inexperienced observers of nature may be reminded of the fact that we have unfortunately become unable either hygienically or aesthetically to experience or observe the ideal beauty and health of man living under perfectly natural conditions. If there is pleasure to be derived from the beautiful, then displeasure must be felt by an aesthetic eye in looking upon the disharmony of shape and color which in turn leads to a certain degree to the recognition of a pathological condition.

Let us return to our subject. We know that medical science has no answer for baldness, and that cosmetics and hair tonic treatments have yet to produce even a single new hair.

I agree with Prof. Dr. Jaeger who called human hair the odor regulator of the body, conductors for perspiration. Everybody knows that we perspire first on the head and under the arms and that, especially on sick people, a disagreeable odor is noted. Dr. Jaeger somewhere calls disease 'stench'.

This, with exceptions of course, seems to me correct in so far as I have come to conclude on the basis of many years' observation and experiments that all diseases have fundamentally the same uniform causes: Disease is the result of a process of fermentation and decay of body substances or of food surpluses which have accumulated in the course of time especially in the digestive organs and which become a form of mucus matter. In other words we are concerned here with the chemical decomposition, the decay of cellular albumen. As is well known, this process is accompanied by stench, while nature sees to it that all creation of new life is accompanied by an abundance of fragrance (blossom time of trees and flowers). Man in perfect health should therefore give off a smell of fragrance, particularly through his hair. Poets speak of comparing man with a flower and they praise the fragrance of a lovely woman's hair. I therefore consider human hair as having extremely important and useful functions.

Hair not only serves to protect us and to keep us warm, but has a highly interesting and useful task of regulating the body odors of healthy and sick alike. A close observation of people will enable the more knowledgeable and the amateur with a keen nose to gain insight into a person's qualities and also help him draw conclusions as to the state of health or sickness of an individual. Before a doctor has sometimes recognized digestive troubles with the aid of microscopes and test tubes, a quack might have become aware of the internal process of decay, i.e. the sickness, with the simple help of hair diagnosis. Why, there are many people today who seemingly youthful and radiant with good health

do nevertheless have constant bad breath and are
wondering why their hair is falling out. With this
observation I have arrived at a vital point of my
experiments and research.

First one more word about getting gray hair. It has
been established that in hair which has become
gray the contents of air has increased and I am of
the opinion that this 'air' consists probably of
various kinds of gas, or at least is intermingled with
it. I wish a sagacious chemist would discover the
presence of sulphuric acid in gray hair, for then
fading of the hair color will also have been explained. After all it is a known fact that sulphur-
dioxide bleaches organic substances. It seems certain to me, not only theoretically but also on the
basis of very conclusive experiments on my own
body that the principal cause of baldness is of
internal nature. If, then, the hair acts as an odor
regulator of the body, almost like a chimney
through which the odors are filtered, and all that is
being discharged is stinking gas, very probably
intermingled with sulphur-dioxide, instead of natural, fragrant odors, we must not be surprised
when the hair and its roots suffocate, become pale,
die and fall out. I am confident to have recognized
the cause for baldness and to have shown the true
way for its cure. About ten years ago, when I was
afflicted with chronic inflammation of the kidneys
and suffered from nervous tension, my hair turned
very gray and started to fall out. However, as soon
as I had been cured from this serious disease by a
dietetic treatment, the streaks of gray disappeared
and my hair grew remarkably thick and healthy.

If therefore baldness stems from digestive troubles

and malfunctioning of the metabolism, it follows that it can be remedied only by first alleviating those very causes. On the basis of my discovery I dare say that there is still hope even for the bald heads on whom all the tonics have failed and had to fail. The reason for failure is of course the recognition that the cause is not external and therefore cannot be treated externally. Whoever is losing hair to an alarming degree or whoever is already bald and wishes to regenerate himself, may take my advice. It is understood that there is no general all-round remedy but rather, in line with my whole theory of cure, an individual evaluation and treatment will be necessary in each and every case. This much however is certain, I can guarantee that loss of hair will stop even in serious cases provided my teachings for a proper diet will be adhered to.

Thus all symptoms of aging are latent disease, accumulation of mucus and clogging up of the system with mucus. Anybody who takes to a careful diet of mucusless foods in case of any disease, possibly followed up by a fast, will rid his body of the dead cells which have accumulated there in the course of many years and will not only better his condition but at the same time rejuvenate himself. And whoever rejuvenates himself will simultaneously build up his resistance to disease to a remarkable degree. Nobody seems to believe in this possibility. Yet, each scientific dictionary will tell you that under normal circumstances the natural causes of death should be arteriosclerosis due to a slowed down metabolism, i.e., clogging up of the entire organism, and therefore life ought to end without any disease whatever. This would be the normal situation, but alas, the exception, the disease, has become the rule today.

If everybody lived only on mucusless food from his earliest youth and ate nothing but fruit, it would stand to reason that he could grow neither old nor sick. I have seen people who became so rejuvenated and beautiful after a mucusless diet cure that I almost didn't recognize them. For thousands of years humanity has indulged in dreams and wishful thinking about the fountain of youth and has been looking for it in the stars.

Just think of the amount of money spent on remedies for impotence and sterility, of course all in vain. And yet, it could be so easy to give help at least to some people simply by putting them on a better healthier diet.

We can hardly imagine the beauty and strength with which the paradisiacal 'godlike' man was endowed, what kind of wonderful, strong and clear voice he had! One of the amazing results of my cure is a remarkable improvement in the voice, a strengthening of the vocal cords. Even a lost voice can be reactivated which is eloquent proof indeed of the far reaching effects of my system on the entire human organism. I wish to refer here especially to the tremendous success that the Royal Bavarian Chamber Singer Heinrich Knote, Munich, achieved through a cure under my direction. His voice improved in clarity and beauty to such an extent that the entire musical world was amazed and full of the highest praise.

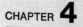

CHAPTER 4

Increasing longevity

In the previous chapters I stated that the reason for disease and aging is the accumulation of mucus in the body. I also proved the possibility of cell regeneration through fasting and fruit diet. Therefore, if man feeds on fruit only all his life, death can be delayed for a long, long time. Fruit eaters, at any rate, have a greater life expectancy than people who indulge in all the wrong foods. Their metabolism works better and, due to their correct diet, less strain is placed on the organs, especially the heart and stomach. It is noteworthy that the heartbeat of a fruit eater, even when he exerts himself physically, is not nearly as high as that of the mucus eater. The energy thus saved daily can be figured out mathematically and proves the increased longevity stated above.

When man dies of a critical injury or disease it is because his heart and brain cease to function. However, what causes these vital organs to stop their activity? In most cases the disease raging in the body will weaken the heart and eventually cause heart failure. Regarding causes for this failure, science has by far not spoken its last word. We can, however, safely say that the clogging up of blood vessels, consequently paralyzing the heart muscle and causing the destruction of the tender heart nerves through constant re-poisoning of the blood, is the final cause of death in all chronic diseases. Likewise, the clogging up of tender blood vessels in the brain and their eventual bursting (apoplexy) as well as any other entire clogging up of vessels result in a standstill of all functions of life, i.e. death. Other secondary causes come into play as well, of course, such as insufficient supply of oxygen in case of lung disease, etc. Science also mentions that an overabundance of white corpuscles will result in death. As we know, this is a disease in itself called leukemia. In plain English this means "white bloodedness", but in my opinion more accurately yet "more mucus than blood". Naturally, many more reasons are given as the cause of death.

I now ask, what is really the killing poison? Modern medical science claims that the bacilli cause most diseases, thus showing that it also has the idea of a common fundamental cause of all diseases, aging and death. Undoubtedly, diseases and their consequence (death) are to a large degree due to the bacilli. My experiments which prove that mucus is the fundamental and main cause differ from the bacillus theory only in that mucus is the nutrient medium for all bacilli.

As we have seen, an abundance of white blood cells, i.e. of white dead mucus, as compared with the red sugar and iron substances, is a menace to life. Red is the color and sweet is the taste of life and love; white or pale is the sign of sickness and mucus building up in the body, a sign of gradual disintegration.

The death struggle is only the last effort of the organism to excrete mucus, a last fight of the still living cells against the dead ones and their deathly poisons. If the white dead cells, i.e. the mucus in the blood, gain the upper hand, clogging up of the blood vessels of the heart occurs. At the same time a chemical transformation, a sudden poisoning of the entire blood supply system takes place and death takes its toll.

part two

CHAPTER 5

Complete instructions for fasting

Most diseases are due to wrong eating habits, incorrect food combinations, acidulous foods and the unnatural nourishment of present day civilization. How to overcome the results of these errors that the majority of us ignorantly inflict upon ourselves will be taught in the following pages.

For thousands of years fasting has been recognized as nature's supreme curative measure. But the art of when, why and how to fast has been with a very few exceptions lost by those living in present day civilization. The body must have good nourishing food is the battle cry of today. But just what is good nourishing food?

The unfortunate sufferers make the rounds of the various schools of therapeutics. They are very often ignorant, grope in the dark and search in vain for the truth. And the most unfortunate part of it all is that they die before they learn the truth.

Evangelists and divine healers have an advantage in that they give Nature a chance.

An overdose of medication, surgery, injections and vaccinations can easily become the offenders of an outraged Nature. And so it resolves itself into a case of "blind leading the blind". And yet, it is so simple to receive instructions from Nature. Watch the animals heal themselves in time of illness without the use of so-called scientific medicine. This then is the supreme secret of Mother Nature's selfhealing.

In the following chapters I will give an indication of the kind of foods, cooked as well as raw, that are necessary to guarantee a properly balanced diet. I will also explain the causes of fermentation and of gas producing foods.

CHAPTER 6

Rational fasting for physical, mental and spiritual rejuvenation

It is significant for our time of degeneration that fasting, by which I mean living without solid and liquid food, is still not fully recognized for its worth by the average man, nor by the orthodox medical doctor as well. Even Naturopathy required a few decades in its development before it turned to Nature's only, universal and omnipotent remedy. It is furthermore significant that fasting is still considered as a 'special' kind of cure, and due to some truly impressive results here and there, it has quite recently become a world-wide fad. Even some experts of the Nature cure have gotten carried away and have drawn up some general rules and prescriptions for fasting, and how to break a fast, regardless of the condition or the disease of the sufferer.

On the other hand, fasting has been quite misrepresented so that the average man actually considers it to be dangerous to miss out on a few meals during sickness for fear that he will starve to death, when in reality he is being cured. He equates fasting and starvation. The medical doctor in general is not without blame for having perpetuated such foolish belief which is quite in contrast to Nature's laws of self-healing and curing.

Whatever goes by the name of "natural treatments" for the elimination of diseased matter and does not at least require some measure of restriction or change in diet, or fasting, is basically disregarding the truth concerning the cause of disease.

Have you ever thought when you were sick what it means to have no appetite? And that wild animals have no doctors, no drug stores, no sanitariums, and no equipment to give them help? Nature teaches us through this example that there is basically only *one* disease, the one caused by overeating and eating of the wrong foods. Therefore, this *one* disease or whatever the many different names man may have given it, can be cured by but *one* remedy, namely by withholding from the body those very substances which normally will bring about disease. In other words, do exactly the opposite of overeating: reduce your intake of foods, improve on your general diet and prepare for some fasting. The reason so many fasting cures, especially those of longer duration, have failed and continue to fail is the ignorance of its proper application and the lack of understanding as to what is going on in the body during a fast. Naturopaths and fasting experts are not always as well aware as they should be in this delicate area. I dare say that possibly there isn't another man in history who has studied, investigated, tested and experimented with fasting as much as I have. As far as I know there is no other specialist at present who could claim to have conducted as many fasting cures even in very severe cases of disease as I have. I set up the first sanitarium in the world

which specialized in fasting combined with the
mucusless diet as an essential prerequisite for my
Mucusless Diet Healing System.* I have furthermore undertaken publicly several fasts for scientific research, lasting from 21 to 24 to 32 days
respectively in demonstration of my method of
healing. The latter test represents the world record
of a fast conducted under strict scientific supervision of government officials.

You therefore know that from my own experiments I have good knowledge of what actually
happens in the body during a fast. Previously I
talked about the body which can be compared in
its mechanism to a machine. Now imagine that this
mechanism, made of a rubber-like material, has
been overworked for years due to high intake of
food, thereby expanding the tissues and vessels to
accommodate the high proportion of residues.
Hence the continuously overburdened organism
puts unusual pressure on the blood and the tissues.
As soon as you stop eating, this excessive pressure
is rapidly relieved, the highly over-expanded blood
vessels and tissues relax, blood becomes more
concentrated and superfluous water is eliminated.
This process continues for a few days during which
you may feel quite all right, but as the vessels
contract, the mucus which lines their inner walls
creates an obstruction for the blood circulation in
as much as the passage becomes very narrow.
Therefore the blood must in the process of its

* Mucusless Diet Healing System available from this publisher $1.95
plus 35 cents mailing and handling cost.

circulation through the body, especially in the tissues, circumvent, dissolve and carry with it the mucus and its poisonous substances for eventual elimination through the kidneys.

During their fast the primary immediate obstructions caused by wrong and too much eating are eliminated first. This results in your feeling relatively good, or possibly even better than when eating. However when—as previously explained—the blood stream begins to carry with it some of the loosened mucus matter from the obstructed passages, then you feel miserable. You and everybody else blame this feeling on the lack of food which is true but only to the extent that this whole cleansing process is set into motion by the absence of new food. The next day for sure you can notice mucus matter in the urine. Once the waste products have been eliminated from the circulation you will undoubtedly feel fine, even stronger than ever before. It is a well known fact that a faster can feel better and is actually stronger on the twentieth day of his fast than on the fifth or sixth day. Certainly ample proof that vitality does not depend primarily on food but rather on an unobstructed circulation. (See Lesson 5 of my Mucusless Diet Healing System). The smaller the amount of obstruction the greater the air pressure and consequently more vitality.

The above explanations will have given you an insight into the nature of a fasting cure. At first it is a negative proposition to relieve the body of direct obstruction by abstaining from solid foods. Secondly it is a mechanical process by means of the contracting tissues and vessels whereby mucus matter is freed and causes friction and obstruction in the circulation.

The following are examples of strength gained during a fast: One of my first fasters, a relatively healthy vegetarian, walked 45 miles in the mountains on his 24th fasting day.

After a ten day fast a friend fifteen years younger and I undertook a 56 hour walk.

A German physician, a specialist in fasting cures, published a pamphlet entitled "Fasting increases Vitality". He obtained the same results as I did but he didn't discover the reasons for this extraordinary increase in vitality which remained a mystery to him.

If you drink only water during a fast the human mechanism cleanses itself in a similar fashion as if you were to squeeze out a dirty sponge, but the dirt in this instance is sticky mucus in many cases intermingled with pus and drugs. It will remain in the blood circulation until it is so thoroughly dissolved that it can eventually pass through the kidneys to the infinite relief of the body and its owner.

CHAPTER 7

Building a perfect body thru fasting

As long as the waste is in the circulation you feel miserable during a fast; as soon as it is thru the kidneys you feel fine. Two or three days later and the same process repeats itself. This will explain why conditions change so often during a fast, why it is possible for you to feel unusually better and stronger on the twentieth than on the fifth day, for instance.

As this entire cleansing process (thru continued contracting of the tissues—becoming lean) has to be done by and with the original old blood composition of the patient, a long fast, especially a too long a fast, would be criminal if the sick organism is too greatly clogged up by waste. Fasters who died from too long a fast did not die from lack of food but died from their own waste, i.e. they actually suffocated. More clearly expressed: The immediate cause of death is not a lack of vital substances in the blood but too much obstruction. Obstruction becomes as great as or even greater than air pressure and, therefore, the body mechanism is "deadlocked."

FASTERS SHOULD DRINK LEMON JUICE EITHER UNSUGARED OR WITH A TRACE OF

HONEY OR BROWN SUGAR FOR LOOSENING
AND THINNING THE MUCUS IN THE CIRCU-
LATION. Lemon juice and fruit acids of all kinds
neutralize the stickiness of mucus and pus. Anyone
who has ever taken medication or drugs has to be
very careful when he takes his first fast. As the
drugs leave residues which are stored up in the
body like the waste from food (I saw patients
eliminate drugs they had taken as long as forty
years ago), his condition might easily become
serious or even dangerous when these poisons enter
the circulation. Palpitation of the heart, headaches,
nervousness and especially sleeplessness may occur.
Everybody, and especially doctors, blame these
symptoms on the fast.

How Long Should One Fast?

Nature answers this question in the animal kingdom with a certain cruelty: "fast until you are
either healed or dead." In my estimation 50 to
60% of the so-called healthy men of today and 80
to 90% of the seriously chronic sick would die
from their latent diseases if they submitted to a
long fast.

How long one should fast cannot be determined in
advance, even in cases where the condition of the
patient is known. When and how to break the fast
is determined by noting carefully how conditions
change during the fast. It should definitely be
broken as soon as you notice that the obstruction
in the circulation is becoming too great and that
the blood needs new vital substances to resist and

neutralize the poisons. It is wrong to assume the attitude: "the longer you fast the better the cure" and you may now readily understand why.

Man is the sickest animal on earth in that no other animal has violated the laws of eating as much as man and no other animal eats as wrongly as man. Here is where human intelligence can correctively assist in the self-healing process by the following adjustments which embrace the Mucusless Diet Healing System:

> 1. Prepare for an easier fast by gradually changing your diet toward a mucusless diet and by using laxatives and enemas.
> 2. In between fasts eat nothing but a cleansing mucus-poor and mucusless diet.
> 3. Be particularly careful if you have been using drugs, especially those containing mercury, salpetre or oxide of silver which is prominent in drugs taken for venereal diseases. Before going on a fast, be sure to allow your body to adjust VERY GRAD-UALLY to a preparatory diet.

An "expert's" suggestion to fast until the tongue is clean has had some grave consequences with "fanatical" fasters who heeded it. I personally know of one case which resulted in death and you may be surprised when I tell you that I had to cure patients from the ill-effects of too long a fast. The reason will be clear later.

In spite of the above, every cure, and especially

every diet cure, should start with a two or three day fast. Every patient can do this without any harm, regardless of how seriously sick he may be. First a laxative and then an enema daily makes it easier as well as harmless.

HOW TO BREAK A FAST

It is of utmost importance to know how to break a fast, i.e. what to eat after a fast. This depends, of course, entirely upon the condition of the patient and to a great extent on the length of the fast. The following two examples of extreme cases, both of which ended fatally not from the fast but from the first wrong meal, were chosen to demonstrate just why this knowledge is so important.

A one-sided meat eater suffering from diabetes broke his fast, which lasted about a week, by eating dates and died. A man of over 60 years of age fasted twenty-eight days. After his first meal of vegetarian food (mainly boiled potatoes), his condition became so serious that an operation had to be performed. It showed that in the contracted intestines passage of the potatoes had been blocked by thick sticky mucus which was so strong that a piece had to be cut off. The patient died shortly after the operation.

The example of the meat eater shows that when the terrible poisons, loosened in the stomach during the fast, mixed with the concentrated fruit sugar of the dates such a great fermentation (car-

bonic acid gases and other poisons) set in that the
patient could not stand the shock. In this case, it
would have been advisable to break the fast as
follows: first a harmless herbal laxative, later raw
and cooked starchless vegetable, a piece of rough
bran bread toast. Sauerkraut is also to be recommended. Since the patient was not prepared for the
fast by a gradual transition diet, he as a meat eater
should have had no fruit for a long time after the
fast.

As to the second example, the patient fasted
entirely too long for a man of his age and, again, he
was not properly prepared for the fast.

These two very instructive examples show how
individualized the advice on how to break a fast
has to be and that it would be wrong to make a
hard and fast rule. What can be said in general,
however, and what I teach is new and different
from the average fasting experts, I have summa-
rized as "IMPORTANT RULES FOR THE FAST-
ER TO BE CAREFULLY STUDIED AND MEM-
ORIZED."

> 1 - After a fast, do not eat particularly
> nourishing food, this would be a mistake.
> All meals for a few days after the fast
> should have a laxative effect.

> 2 - The sooner the first meal passes thru
> the body the more efficiently it clears
> away the loosened mucus and poisons in
> the stomach and intestines.

3 - If no good stool is experienced after two or three hours after the first meal, help with laxatives and enemas. Whenever I fasted I always had a good bowel movement at least one hour after eating and at once felt fine. After breaking a long fast, I spent more time the following night on the toilet than in bed, and that was as it should be.

While sojourning in Italy many years ago, I drank about two quarts of fresh grape juice after a fast and instantly experienced a watery diarrhea of foaming mucus. Almost immediately after that, I had a feeling of such unusual strength that I easily performed the knee bending and arm stretching exercises 326 times. This thorough cleansing of the body, i.e. removal of all obstruction, which took place after a fast of a few days, increased my vitality at once! You will have to experience a similar sensation to believe me and you will then agree with my formula: vitality equals strength after all obstruction in the body has been cleared away. And you will also realize the absurdity of making up scientifically nourishing menus for health and strength after a fast.

4 - The longer the fast the more efficiently will the bowels perform after the first meal.

5 - The best laxative food after a fast is fresh sweet fruit, especially cherries and grapes or slightly soaked or stewed prunes. However only people who have lived for a certain time on mucusless or at least mucus-poor food, i.e. a transition diet, are permitted fruit after a fast. As we have seen before, absolutely no fruit for meat eaters!

6 - Generally speaking, it is advisable to break the fast with raw and cooked starchless vegetable, stewed spinach for example, has an especially good effect.

7 - If the first meal does not cause any unpleasantness, you may eat as much as you can. Eating only a small quantity of food for the first 2 or 3 days after the fast without experiencing a bowel movement due to the small amount of food taken in (another wrong advice given by "experts") is dangerous.

8 - If you prepared properly for the fast and can start eating fruit after breaking the fast and you have no bowel movement after about an hour, then eat more fruit or a vegetable meal as suggested above. At any rate, eat until you experience a good stool that will relieve you of the waste accumulated during the fast.

Rules During the Fast

1. Clean the lower intestines as well as you can with enemas at least every other day.

2. Before starting a longer fast prepare for it and take a laxative occasionally and definitely the day before you start the fast.

3. It is important that you get as much fresh air as possible therefore remain outdoors as much as you can during the day and keep windows open at night.

4. If you feel strong enough, go for a walk or do some light physical work. If tired and weak, rest and sleep as much as you can.

5. On days when you feel weak—you will experience such days especially when the waste is in the circulation—your sleep may be restless and disturbed and you may have bad dreams. This is caused by the poisons passing thru the brain.

If doubt and loss of faith in the fasting cure will arise in your mind then take this lesson and read it over and over again, as well as the other fasting chapters. Also, don't forget that you are lying on "Nature's operating table", the most wonderful of all operations that could be performed and without surgery!

However, if any extraordinary sensation occurs due to the poisons now in circulation, take an enema at once, lie down and if necessary break the fast. Raw and cooked starchless vegetables such as Sauerkraut or stewed spinach are recommended.

6. Whenever you have rested for a while, get up slowly because otherwise you may become dizzy and that is a very unpleasant and somewhat scary experience. It caused me considerable fear in the beginning and I know of a number of people who gave up on fasting altogether when they experienced this sensation, although it is not serious and is nothing to worry about.

FASTING DRINKS

Many "fanatic" fasters drink nothing but water thinking that it is best to avoid any trace of food whatsoever. I CONSIDER A LIGHT LEMONADE WITH A LITTLE HONEY OR BROWN SUGAR OR A LITTLE FRUIT JUICE THE BEST. Drink as often as you feel like it, but in general no more than 2 or 3 quarts a day. The less you drink the more aggressively the fast works.

During a longer fast you should, as a change, drink also vegetable juice made from raw starchless vegetables (raw tomato juice, etc. for example). If fruit juice, orange juice for instance, is used exclusively during a longer fast you have to be extremely careful because the fruit juices may cause the poisons to become loosened too rapidly without causing a bowel movement. I know of a number of such fruit and fruit juice fasts which failed completely because too much mucus and all of the poisons loosened too quickly at the same time. Then this waste, once in the circulation, disturbs all the organs and can only be eliminated thru the circulation with the aid of bowel movements.

MORNING FAST OR NON-BREAKFAST PLAN

The worst of all eating habits nowadays is to stuff the stomach with food early in the morning. In European countries, except in England, no one has a regular meal for breakfast, just a beverage of some kind and bread.

The one time that man does not eat for a period of 10 to 12 hours is while he is asleep, and as soon as the stomach is free from food, the body starts the elimination process of the accumulated waste. Therefore, people feel miserable and have a coated tongue upon waking up. They have no appetite at all yet they crave food and feel better after breakfast.—Why?

This is a mystery that has puzzled all "experts". They believe that it is the nourishing quality in the food that makes us feel better. I discovered, however, that as soon as you refill the stomach with food THE PROCESS OF ELIMINATING THE ACCUMULATED WASTE—which, as I described, is somewhat unpleasant—IS STOPPED and therefore you feel better! I think that my discovery undoubtedly explains also why eating became a habit and is no longer what nature intended it to be, i.e., a satisfaction, a compensation of nature's need for food.

This habit of eating proves the saying I coined long ago: "Life is a tragedy of nutrition". The more waste man accumulates the more he must eat in order to stop the elimination of waste. I had patients who had to eat several times during the night to be able to sleep again. In other words, they had to put food into their stomachs to avoid the digestion of mucus and poisons.

Short Fasts And The Non-Breakfast Plan

As we have seen, upon awakening you perhaps feel fine but instead of getting up you remain in bed and fall asleep again, have a bad dream and actually feel miserable upon awakening the second time. As soon as you get up, walk around or do something, the body is in an entirely different condition than during the sleep and the process of eliminating waste is slowed down, the energy being used elsewhere.

If you skip breakfast every morning you will probably experience some harmless sensations such as headaches for the first one or two days. Thereafter you will feel much better, work better, and enjoy your luncheon better than ever. Hundreds of severe cases have been cured by the Non-Breakfast Plan alone, proving that the habit of eating a full breakfast meal is the worst of all.

You may enjoy the same beverage for breakfast

that you are accustomed to. If you crave coffee
continue to drink coffee, but abstain definitely
from SOLID FOOD! Later on, replace the coffee
with a warm vegetable juice and still later change
to lemonade. This change should be made very
gradually.

THE 24 HOUR FAST, OR ONE MEAL A DAY PLAN

The benefits to be derived from the breakfast fast
can be even further improved by the 24 hour fast.
It is also a good preliminary step to the longer fasts
necessary to cure the more severe cases of chronic
disease. The best time to eat is 3 or 4 o'clock in the
afternoon. If you are on the mucusless or transition diet, start with fruits (fruits should always be
eaten first) and about 15 or 20 minutes later eat
the vegetables; but all should be eaten within an
hour so that it is to say, one meal.

FASTING WHEN USED IN CONNECTION WITH THE MUCUSLESS DIET HEALING SYSTEM

As I have stated before I am no longer in favour of
long fasts. In fact it may become criminal to let a
patient fast for 30 or 40 days on water for this
would cause the contracting tissues and vessels to
excrete more and more mucus which intermingled
with residues from previously taken dangerous
drugs etc. could actually result in self-poisoning if
no new vital food elements are added to the body.

No one can stand a fast of that kind without harm to his strength.

If fasting is to be used at all, then start at first with the non-breakfast plan, subsequently follow the 24 hour fast for a while, then gradually increase the fast to 3, 4 or 5 days interspersed with 1, 2, 3, or 4 days of mucusless diet. In this way the body is simultaneously rebuilt and supplied with the best nourishment found only in mucusless foods.

Through such intermittent fasts the blood is gradually improved and regenerated and can more easily withstand the poisons and waste. It is at the same time better equipped to dissolve and eliminate these many years old deposits which are loosened up by the fast, deposits that no doctor ever thought existed and that no one has known how to remove.

These are the merits of the invaluable mucusless diet healing system of which fasting is an essential feature.

FASTING IN CASES OF ACUTE DISEASE

"Hunger cures—Miracle cures" was the title of the first fasting book I ever read. It related the experiences of a country doctor who stated: "No acute feverish disease need end in death provided Nature's instinctive command to stop eating thru lack of appetite is obeyed".

It is insane for instance to give food to a patient who suffers from pneumonia accompanied by high temperatures. A 'cold' having caused an unusual contraction of the lung tissues results in a loosening and propelling of some of the mucus deposits into the circulation. This produces an unusual friction: fever, and it would aggravate the patients condition even more if solid foods, meat broth etc. were given to him resulting in more fuel added to the already overheated human engine. The lives of many of the pneumonia patients could have been saved if only they had been given enemas, laxatives, cool lemonade and some exposure to fresh air in their rooms. However, the medical profession is sometimes very reluctant to follow new directions.

SPIRITUAL REBIRTH THRU THE SUPERIOR FAST

All experts, except myself, believe that you live on your reserves during a fast. You, however, know now, that what is called metabolism is simply the elimination of waste.

The Muslim or Hindu fakir, the greatest religious ascetic and faster in the world today, is usually very slender. I learned that the more thoroughly cleansed the body is the easier it is to fast and the longer you can stand it. In other words, when you are free from all waste and poisons, and when no solid foods are taken, then the human body functions for the first time in its life without encountering obstructions. The elasticity of the entire tissue system and of the internal organs, especially of the spongy lungs, responds to a single intake of breath with an entirely different vibration and an efficiency never known before. You ascend into a higher state of physical, mental and spiritual being. I call that the "Superior Fast".

When you eat only the foods which I recommend, then your blood will be regenerated miraculously and your mind will function extremely well. Your former life will take on the appearance of a dream, and for the first time in your existence your conscience awakens to a real self-consciousness.

Your mind, your thinking, your ideals, your aspirations and your philosophy will change fundamentally for the better. Your soul will shout with joy and triumph over all misery of life. For the first time you will feel a vibration of vitality thru your body like a slight electric current that shakes you delightfully.

You will realize that fasting and superior fasting (and not volumes of psychology and philosophy) are the real and only key to a superior life; to the revelation of a superior spiritual world.

CHAPTER 8

Conclusion

While I have conducted thousands of fasting cures, any number of people have been helped by simply changing their dietary habits. However, a change made too rapidly may become dangerous and to relieve and avoid any disturbance of health I suggest you follow my transition diet.

Changing from a meat diet to a strictly vegetarian or fruit diet always results in a more vigorous feeling for the first few days, then weakness, great fatigue, possibly headaches and palpitation of the heart set in. Fruit being the only natural food, it loosens and dissolves the mucus and poison which are eliminated by the blood stream and the dead decayed tissues are pushed aside to make room for the new living food substances. This elimination process causes some discomfort and unless you are thoroughly convinced of the efficacy of the natural diet, your friends will dissuade you from further attempts to cleanse the body. In fact, they will urge you to interrupt this cleansing process in order to save you from what they believe will ruin your health. Soon you will become lean, the face will appear haggard and drawn and a general feeling of depression may overtake you. This then is the healing crisis which, once overcome, will result in unexpected good health.

I divide all food into the following two kinds:

1. Mucus-forming food, i.e. meat, eggs, fats, milk and all by-products of milk, dried beans, dried peas, lentils and ALL STARCHY FOODS.

2. Non-mucus forming food, i.e. all green vegetable and all kinds of fruit. However, certain types of vegetable and fruit contain some starch and therefore should be given second place.

Begin the transition period by avoiding mucus-forming food as much as possible. After having conditioned your body, the next step toward health is the MUCUSLESS DIET which is a combination of starchless vegetable and fruit. With the help of this transition diet and some knowledge by the individual to choose and combine rightly, the greatest and most important truth of life is revealed to him.

The so-called strength which we experience after having eaten meat is nothing but a stimulation, for there is no nourishment for man in meat. In fact, the waste products of meat, fatty plaque-shaped particles, are deposited on the walls of the blood vessels where in time they form a thick lining, calcify and thus contribute to the hardening of the arteries. This hardening of the arteries, in many cases resulting in high blood pressure, is the chief cause of heart attacks and diseases of senility. Tests on animals have already shown that meat-eating animals will die if fed on cooked meat alone. And rats soon die if kept on a diet of white flour.

My mucus theory has been recognized more and more. It has passed all tests successfully and today has established that: NATURAL TREATMENT AND DIET IS THE MOST PERFECT AND SUCCESSFUL SYSTEM OF HEALING KNOWN. Thru my Rational Fasting and the Mucusless Diet Healing System suffering mankind now has the means of not only relieving but PREVENTING disease. And my most fervent hope is that it will bring better health and happiness to all mankind.

APPENDIX

Following are a series of seven
individual essays written by
Professor Arnold Ehret.
They have been assembled and published
here to provide a deeper understanding
of the author's basic concept.

My Mucusless Diet and Naturopathy

Professor Ehret, having been sponsored by Dr. Benedict Lust, "The Father of Naturopathy", observed the inter-relationship between his system and that of his patron. He found them in complete harmony and in this article, never before published, explains how they should be combined.

When I first brought out my "Muscus-forming" diet as the fundamental cause of all disease, and my "Mucusless" diet as its only cure, it created great discussion, even in the ranks of Naturopathy. A little later, a professor of medicine advised all physicians to read this book, "Rational Fasting", in which these diets are described. In treating less than twenty cases (my first ones) I observed that every one eliminated mucus. I have since proven this fact by over two thousand cases. If a so-called healthy person is treated with proper elimination, fasting, diet, etc., the urine will show mucus. Standard analysis books state that under a microscope the atoms of mucus and pus cannot be told apart.

Advanced Naturopaths, but not very many, know there is really but one disease, internal impurity, caused by unusable food elements. These impurities are principally from mucus-forming foods, and are the sticky, pasty, and slimey substance, called *mucus*.

Isn't it high time that Naturopaths take up this advanced truth and system and show by their marvelous success its superiority over the present theories of the cause of disease and drug treatment. Should not Naturopaths show results better than the ordinary "cures" (which are but reliefs) of complete cures and become examples, themselves, of Superb Health, examples of perfect immunity from Disease, even examples like myself, of proven immunity and of superb health?

This is "Paradise Health" and only possible by a mucusless diet and rightly conducted fasting. We now know that wrong and too much food is the *cause* of all disease, and its *only* complete cure is by right diet and fasting, Nature's own methods. Even animals adopt fasting when injured or diseased, by instinct. This proves that Nature has only one diagnosis and only one disease, that of internal impurity. Why spend so much time and labor on diagnosis in Naturopathy, Eye diagnosis, etc? Why so little attention paid to right diet and fasting? First, because the right diet for producing vital energy, which we have discovered, is not generally known; second, that fasts have been so crudely conducted; and third, that diet and fasting have not been properly combined. As nature cures all diseases by fasting, it *must* be that *eating* is the *cause* of them.

Why so little attention given to dietetics? Why such a quarrel and such confusion about diet? Why is a fruit or a mucusless diet so little used? Why have fruit, vegetables, etc., so little credit for their vital energy producing qualities? The very evident reasons are: First, because they are not generally known, or considered only as relishes or ornaments to a table or as a help to elimination, and *not* as they are, superior energy producers. Second, that it is absolutely necessary to use them with a diet with some mucus or "mucus-poor" as a transition diet in successful fasting. Third, they are evidently instituted and scientifically and practically demonstrated. It is the *only* diet that can produce what we have rightly named, Paradise Health.

Disease is a beneficial result of the natural and intelligent efforts of the vital energy of the body to cleanse it of all impurities. These impurities we call mucus, but it includes all other toxic mixtures, mucus being its most plentiful kind. Nature can accomplish the cleansing *only* if you don't eat, and for this reason shuts down the appetite, even in a simple cold. Why do not people reduce their food or fast when Nature's law lessens or stops the desire for food? Because they do not understand that the weakness which accompanies loss of appetite is a curative process, the impurities being eliminated by the blood stream. Man is more degenerated than animals in eating or curing of disease.

Civilization has brought a greater cleanliness on the outside of the body, but an *awful* uncleanliness inside. No one can imagine or realize this until he has treated some hundreds of patients by fasting and diet, as I have. No animal on earth is so full of undigested, fermented and decayed foodstuffs from overeating and unnatural food as so-called civilized man. If any one starts a fruit or mucusless diet or a fast, without intelligent knowledge of how to prepare for them, the decayed material—largely mucus—is loosened up all over the system, enters the blood stream, causing extreme weakness which he does not understand, and this may put his life in danger.

A prominent non-Naturopathic practitioner is erroneously advising increased eating, even of meat, before starting a fast; while just the opposite course is the right one. When preparing or "training" for my 49-day fast, under strict observation, I lived on a strictly mucusless diet for over two years and took short fasts meanwhile. The "master" of fasting is the East Indian Fakir, whose body is only skin and bones. There is no greater error than in believing that the tissue of the body "breaks down" during a fast, or eats itself, becomes a "cannibal," as a prominent Sanitarium man declares.

My experience is that fleshy persons or those highly encumbered with mucus are distressed the most by a fast. The loosened up mucus gets into the blood stream causing extreme weakness sooner, and the amount is so much larger that the weak period lasts much longer before the increased strength comes. These are the dangerous cases instead of the thin persons, whose poisonous encumbrance is much less. The fleshy ones are like pneumonia patients, suffocated (choked) by their own poisonous mucus or auto-intoxication. Not a single faster dies or has died from starvation, but from his own self-poisoning, often enhanced by wrong diet as the fast ends. Orange juice is often advised in this country, which is right in some cases, but for a heavily encumbered or fleshy patient it is quite dangerous. Orange juice is an ideal food, but when mixed with the awful poisonous mixture in the stomach of the faster, it adds to the quickness with which it is taken up by the blood, and is likely to harm the patient.

There is much to be learned about fasting and a mucusless diet, simple as it looks to a layman, for no two cases need just the same preparatory diet or length of fast, should be supervised by one of experience. The mucusless diet preparation and short fasts, to commence with, are the "Master Keys" to Superb Health for every one.

To change from the "awful" diet of civilization, at once, without a good knowledge of the mucusless diet, is for most persons dangerous. The so-called healthy persons of today do not know the amount of auto-poisonous encumbrance they have acquired.

This is the reason why a right diet and fasting are so much misunderstood and wrongly used by both practitioner and laymen. Naturopaths must know how to prepare for themselves and conduct, and finish a fast, with the right diet for each step, before taking a patient, *then* they have the *only* and *absolute* agencies for prevention of disease and a perfect cure.

The diet of civilization has brought mankind into an awful state of diseased conditions and epidemics. Centenarians are getting as scarce as diamonds. No one is dying a natural death, without disease; and these results are due to ignorance and the dominating erroneous teaching and practice of the drug cults.

It is so self-evident that the present diet of the civilized countries, of wrong and too much food, is the fundamental factor and cause of all present ailments, that it is with the same self-evidence as a specially educated and prepared expert that I present the mucusless diet and scientifically conducted fasting as the *only* reasonable, simple, natural and infallible "remedies" to bring mankind back to a better and a Paradise-like Health, which it once enjoyed. I have completely cured many of the so-called incurable cases during my 15 years of experience in Europe (10 in conducting a Sanitarium), even those that were not curable by the physical treatments of Physiotherapy. When I developed the mucusless diet and combined it with my improved fasting methods as a *system*, and used them as primary remedies, I was not only able to bring patients back to ordinary health, but to a condition of tremendous efficiency and endurance. Also not only immunity from ailments, but to what we have appropriately named, *paradise health*; which means that *all* the faculties of the body are improved. I proved all of these points in my own person, first, and subsequently successfully in others.

To secure these in one's self or in patients, there must be a slow change from the wrong to the mucusless diet, by a transition diet which I have described in my book, "Muscusless Diet Healing System". The transition diet must be of foods with less mucus—"mucus-poor"—and advised according to the age, condition, business, climate and season of the year, in each case. The first diet used should be changed, according to the reaction, after a short trial, and slowly advanced towards the mucusless diet, until the mucus is loosened and dissolved, and the system so cleansed that a short fast can be taken, and then these can be progressed in length until the desired cleansing is accomplished.

I have described in detail the ideal result of the mucusless diet and improved methods of fasting in this book. The mucusless diet of a more or less degree can be combined with moderate physical applications of Naturopathy with great success. For Naturopathy to grow in favor and to assist in combating wrong methods, it must show a greater degree of success. It must not be satisfied with a temporary relief (an anesthetic will give that), but must bring about a complete cure. I have had many patients that have been benefited by Naturopathic treatments, but not perfectly cured or made immune. If we shall finally get Medical Freedom and a free field for Drugless Healing, it *must* be by a

greater success in curing, and not wholly by litera-
ture and arguments. This surely can be done by
adopting the agencies described, and the Mucusless
Diet is the "Master Key" to it. Of itself alone it
brings much greater success, but in combination
with improved methods the results are marvelous,
and many pronounce them "miraculous."

The Mucusless Diet Healing System

While he was actively engaged in teaching his system in California, Professor Ehret was invited to submit a paper to be read at the 24th Annual Convention of the American Naturopathic Association by its president, Dr. Benedict Lust. This important paper, read to the delegates September 24, 1920 at the Hotel Commodore in New York City is now disclosed for the first time below.

Ladies and Gentlemen:

It has been suggested that I send a short sketch of my System to be read at this convention, and I am well pleased to comply with the suggestion.

Since the commencement of the Drugless Natural Healing or Naturopathic movement, it has been accepted that disease, regardless of its symptoms, consists of a constitutional encumbrance of a material generally known as foreign matter. Consequently, natural healing consists of methods of treatment to eliminate this disease producing material, and to stop the source of it. It is self-evident what this disease producing material comes from, and is the unusable residue of the food eaten, either from too much or from the injurious kinds or from both.

Naturopathy has paid a certain attention to diet regulation but has not recognized that in food were the basic and fundamental principles and elements of both health and disease. In other words the science of Drugless Healing has not yet explained fully enough that the foundational cause of disease, this foreign material, is the undigested, uneliminated and decayed food elements from wrong and too much eating. It is consequently most important, reasonable and clearly seen, that the main factor of drugless healing should consist of dietetics, and this includes intelligently conducted fasting, especially if overeating is the main cause of the patient's disease.

It is an "open secret" that diet is the weak point of chiropractic physicians, because the science of drugless healing lacks a dietetic system that is based upon scientific and fundamental principles and facts and complete enough to be used in every diseased condition. The "Mucusless Diet Healing System" fulfills these two claims completely, for it has proven itself true in my practice in Europe and in this country during a period of over 15 years, as the main factor of healing. It works identically the same in the human body as instinctive self-healing does in the animal. This proves beyond question that it is the only natural healing process of the body itself. This system is based upon my mucus theory—now a well proven fact—and makes plain the former mysteries of every kind of disease. The disease producing material is a partially digested decaying semi-liquid mostly, and in this condition is generally known as mucus. It is easily proven and demonstrated that everyone living on a mixed diet or a starchy vegetarian one, has a more or less clogged up system with mucus, whether sick or not. This foundation cause of every disease is going on from childhood and even before, if animal flesh and animal food products, fats and starchy foods are eaten. It has long been recognized by students and scientists that these foods are not suitable for mankind, as the larger portion cannot be digested fully, but are acted on by the gastric juices making a toxic mucus which decays, ferments, produces gas, acidosis and many kinds of toxins, and this has a sticky and gluey condition and clogs the circulation, so that the body needs a shock like a "cold" to start the elimination of a portion of it. If physical treatments are resorted to, they can only eliminate a portion as long as the supply is not stopped by a change from the mucus forming foods and over-eating is not made. Consequently it is reasonable, natural and self-evident that the disease producing must be stopped if you will have complete success from physical treatments.

Fasting and eating less is the only check on over-eating, and non-mucus forming foods *must* replace mucus forming, disease producing ones. I did not invent or originate fasting or the use of a fruit or improved diet, for those were well known and used long ago as good factors of Naturopathy, but what I did do was to originate an entirely new system of combining them as a systematic healing method, naming it the "Mucusless Diet Healing System", after my "mucus theory" had become a well proven fact as being the largest factor of the fundamental cause of every diseased condition. Neither fasting or the fruit diet has been used in

strict accordance with the condition of the patient,
but to combine them as a "Systematic Cleansing"
the success is remarkable and satisfactory.

The great difference between a diet of healing and
a diet of nourishment seems to be almost unknown
to both practitioners and laymen. Fruit is the ideal,
practical and natural diet of mankind, for nourishment, but the Mucusless Diet is a diet of healing
and consists of raw and cooked fruits, starchless
and leafy vegetables and mucus poor cereals specially prepared. A special or medical diagnosis is
not necessary, nor the local name of the disease,
but the amount of encumbrance of mucus and the
activity of its toxins is of the first importance, and
then, the degree to which the individual's encumbrance has affected his vital energy. Whether the
patient is able to labor and desires to do so, or
whether he is more seriously incapacitated depends
on the speed of the elimination, and upon this depends the degree of weakness and disturbing sensations as the cure proceeds and which can be readily
controlled and regulated.

The toxins of the mucus are chemically lowering
the action of the nerve and muscular systems; and
to see how these conditions affect the organic
functions and impair the vitality, in each individual
case, is the diagnosis.

It is an erroneous idea that only the blood is
affected, is unclean, full of mucus and its toxins,
for the entire body in its deepest tissues have it
stored up. The amount of it is much more than

expected, consequently when it is being dissolved and loosened up by the mucusless diet, care must be taken not to do it too rapidly nor too much, for that clogs the excretory system, impairing the vitality which is already weakened, causing a serious condition; even death can occur. This is important and explains why long fasts or fasts without proper preparation and radical fruit diet attempts to cure, often fail. My diagnosis is a conclusion from my knowledge of the aforementioned points, together with the general appearance of the individual, as to how rapidly he can stand the dissolving of his stored-up mucus, and then advise a transition diet that will make a gradual change from his mucus forming foods to the full action of the mucusless diet. As soon as the greater part of the mucus "deposit" is dissolved and eliminated, a strict mucusless diet is advisable and if necessary can be combined with longer or shorter fasts according to the patient's condition.

Special attention must be given to the bowel movements, as they are the main organs of waste elimination. Artificial means can be used temporarily, from above and below, but the mucusless diet is the only thorough and perfect cleanser that dissolves the dried mucus which sticks to the inner walls of the intestines and colon; and also furnishes the blood with the proper elements that dissolve the mucus that is stored in the walls of the alimentary canal and which stops the peristaltic action of it. To do this is its crowning action in the cure of constipation, and which no other food or laxative has ever succeeded in doing.

The fruits of the mucusless diet furnish the blood with the best nutrient elements as well as dissolvents, and the starchless and leafy vegetables furnish not only the right mineral salts, but the latest finds of the best vitamine foods and "Fat and Water Solubles", "A. B. and C." foods, whatever those mysterious infinitesimal materials are, and their fibres furnish a broom to sweep out the intestinal canal.

The nutritive values of the mucusless diet are superior to those of any other foods. This is well proven by results and by the standard analysis tables when properly interpreted. Their curative and nutritive values were discovered in this country and in Europe at about the same time. I made the discovery during my long experience, tests and experiments resulting in my cure, that the grape-sugar of carbohydrates was the source of vitality and vital energy and *not* the proteins. In 1909 I wrote an article for European health magazines denouncing the metabolic theory and in 1912 learned that Dr. Thomas Powell of Los Angeles had made the same discoveries and was making remarkable cures by using foods containing what he called "Organized Carbon", which is the same food ingredient that develops into the grape-sugar during digestion.

The human body has thousands of feet of small and almost invisible tubes through which the blood circulates like the water in a water motor. If the blood stream contains sticky mucus from wrong eating, the body machine has to run and to work under a continual friction like a car slowed down by applying the brake. This explains the long-existing mystery of weakness and also that of high blood pressure and the high temperature of fever and inflammation. During the process of healing by the Mucusless Diet System, the same friction occurs, because the mucus is dissolved and is taken into the blood stream. But it occurs periodically, because the blood stream cannot carry it all at once.

The up-to-date fasting and fruit diet has been used amateurishly and without any system, and therefore has failed in most cases. This may be the cause why Naturopathy has not yet given full attention to nor fully realized the great value and importance of these two factors of natural healing.

The Mucusless Diet Healing System has been exhaustively tested and its superiority well proven by my success in advising the procedure in thousands of cases, most of them having been pronounced incurable. They consisted of paralysis, blindness, deafness, epilepsy, tuberculosis, diabetes, etc., the *school* in which I acquired the knowledge and graduated from, was in curing my own case of "Bright's Disease". I am not only fully cured physically but the mental is freed from the depressing and hindering effect of the debris from wrong eating and a new life is the result. The only real prevention of disease is found and a new health leading up to the greatest efficiency, strength and endurance. This New Health is not only physical, but mental and spiritual. The mind is not only opened to the highest conception of betterment for self and for all mankind, but there is a spiritual illumination which reveals a possibility of acquirement which is hardly possible to describe.

During the years of my trying to save my own life about 20 years ago, I tried nearly all of the drugless treatments in existence with mostly good reliefs, but would get discouraged after each one when I found I was not cured. Not until I combined fasting with fruits and vegetable diet on my own responsibility and from what I had learned did I accomplish it. In the thousands of cases that I have advised since then I have found that the educational factor is an important one, that the curing is done by Nature's self-healing processes and how they are best assisted. The healing system must be varied and adapted to each individual case. The practitioner should have a practical knowledge of every detail and show in his own person the results of a perfect cure.

If you think that ailing people do not want to miss their "Good Eats", my experience shows that it depends on how sick they are and what they have tried for a "cure", and if they are convinced that our System is the best or *only* one that can really cure them, the change is made readily and the exhilaration of the benefits makes them faithful followers and very earnest advocates.

Very much depends on the advice of the practitioner, how the change during the transition is made, and the food combinations, for a diet that is not enjoyable is not a diet of healing. The Mucus-less Diet changes the taste and takes away the craving for the wrong and stimulating foods to the true nutrients and healthful ones.

The important fact is this: that any chronic disease, which any other kind of treatment cannot cure, is soon benefited by the Mucusless Diet Healing System, and fully healed if the case is curable at all. This System combines satisfactorily with any kind of physical treatments, and by doing this you will get quicker and more satisfactory results, increase your income and help to bring Naturopathy to the victorious success that its natural principles and their application deserve.

Naturopathy has to fight the greatest evil of mankind, which is ignorance, and the diseases which are resultant from it, and also other cults which give temporary relief and finally leave the patient worse than before but claim they are cured. Added to these is the Octopus Medical Trust with its tentacles trying to strangle every kind of healing but its own disastrous and deceiving brand. Its present dominating position makes the outcome problematical unless Naturopathy has greater success. Can we add to it what is proving to be a more complete knowledge of Nature's principles and methods, and bring to mankind its redemption from the diseases and evils of "modern (so-called) civilization" and to Natural Therapy a glorious victory?

The Truth About Human Nourishment and The Conquest of Gluttony

Heretofore unpublished, this revealing article by Professor Ehret provides a concise and practical guide to a fuller understanding of his theory in the battle against what he called "The Tragedy of Nutrition".

While I have directed hundreds of fasting cures, people by the thousands have changed more or less under my direction to a fruit diet. The sudden change to a fruit diet causes disturbances, even in an entirely healthy person, which up to now were completely misunderstood, and which become risky and even dangerous, if conducted incorrectly, or without any directions.

To relieve and to avoid any disturbance of health, to replace the old tidbit enjoyments by new and better ones, I have established a so-called mucus-lean and mucusless diet, during the period of transition to an absolute fruit diet. About this I will enlighten you later. If a meat eater or vegetarian passes suddenly over to a strict fruit diet, the same disturbance will appear as with a fasting person, only with a more slight effect. As a rule, he feels better, more vigorous, until a few days later; then weakness, great fatigue, possibly headache, or palpitation of the heart sets in. At the same time a violent secretion of mucus in the urine, consisting

of phosphates, fat, uric acid and medicines he has
taken or used on his body, takes place.

The ignorance about fruit diet

Fruit, being the only natural food, begins to loosen
and dissolve and to lead away through the circulat-
ing blood the penned up filth and morass of
overfeeding and of wrong useless foods, which
were not fully eliminated.

Any one beginning fruit eating also begins a constitutional healing operation, just like the fasting, he
loses the change of matter balance, not because the
natural food is the *poorest* in albumen, but because
now real living food substances push away the dead
decayed ones, embedded in the tissue of his whole
body.

The breeding conditions for all constitutional and
local disease forms are thus eliminated. His internal
impurity, the filth of gluttony, which are the chief
causes of all diseases, begins to move. The paradisical diet wants to bring him back to the purest purity of paradise, where sickness and disease were not
known.

The human engine has the wonderful power to be
able to clean itself without stopping, at the moment you give it the chance, which means to fast
or eat food poor in albumen. Every disease is the
body's want of this cleaning process, whereby
nature gives the signal by a lack of appetite.

The right understanding for the process of beginning a fruit diet remains hidden to the official world of science, as does the nature of all disease.

Science explains the want of appetite as a change of matter disturbance, caused by not eating enough, and the secretion as pathological symptoms.

The elimination of poison through the circulation of blood causes more or less disturbance of health and produces a burning desire for the old choice morsels. The surrounding friends of the beginning fruit eater are perplexed and shocked, because he grows lean, and urge him to interrupt his internal purification and eat again rich food. The most convinced one becomes an *infidel* and wavers back and forth, and is tempted to give up entirely this badly reputed diet.

Transition diet

I divide all foods into two kinds:

1. Mucus-forming foods.
2. Non-mucus-forming foods.
The first kind are: Meat, eggs, fats, milk, and all products made therefrom, dried beans, dried peas, and dried lentils; further, all starchy foods.

The second kind are: All green vegetables and all kinds of fruit. There are vegetables and fruits which contain more or less starch. The less starch they contain the better they are fitted for food, because starch is nothing but undeveloped grape sugar.

It is best to begin the transition diet with a mucuspoor combination in general, that means, as much as possible mucusless and as little as possible mucus-forming food. The next step is the mucus-less diet, which means a combination of starchless vegetables and fruits.

An elimination of part and a decrease of quantity of mucus-forming foods I call a mucuslean diet. Starch flour products are made more poor of mucus by roasting or toasting. Mucusless diet is the combination of greens, as much as possible, and starchless vegetables and fruit.

With the help of this transition diet and some knowledge by the individual to choose rightly and combine, a relatively healthy person can easily come by degrees to an absolute fruit diet.

Without stumbling and without losing confidence again, the greatest and most important truth of life is revealed to him, the knowledge of the *purest*, *best* and *most perfect*, and at the same time cheapest, form of nourishment. The morbid gluttony disappears by itself, because now he nourishes himself really and rightly and does not fill up, to satisfy his enlarged stomach and stimulate it with substances which, without fail, will lead to disease and final death.

The conquest of gluttony

The cause of gluttony is not to be looked for in mental imbecility, or in a passion to satisfy a perverted appetite. It is a neurasthenic mania, a pathological state of a high, strong and intoxicated nervous system, especially of the organs of digestion, for whose apparent and temporary satisfaction an ever-increasing amount of food-stuffs seems to be necessary. The glutton must, in order to find satisfaction, continually augment the quantities as well as the piquancy of his "eats," just as a drunkard will increase the amount of strong drinks. The glutton will sometimes starve to death because of too much eating; or, what happens more frequently, certain of his organs and ultimately the whole system will refuse to function. Experience teaches us that a voluntary cutting down of the food supply, or temporary fasting, is an annoying hardship for the glutton, as well as of the average man of to-day. His whole mind is possessed by the craze for gluttony and the evil of temptation lies in ambush on all sides. The mere thought of self-denial in eating fills him with horror, and he cannot bear the idea of curtailing the most conventional and the most pleasurable pastime of his miserable existence. If you take away those false pleasures, which to the modern man seem to be indispensable, it is imperative to replace them with those that are natural, healthful, and superior all around. Mankind is entitled to pleasure. I once met an Englishman on his way home from India, who said to me: "We don't know what living is until we have tasted a ripe pineapple fresh from the vine." And I say, and thousands of my followers are saying the same thing: "You must have relished a meal of pure fruit after a fast, if you want to get a faint idea of paradisical enjoyment." The conquest of gluttony will mostly succeed when we are forced into it by circumstances.

But, on the other hand, I am trying to show you a better way, which you will gladly accept after you once have seen the truth which I am trying to present to you.

Gluttony can best be conquered by the substitution of a counter pleasure, which we get through the new diet. Our taste will change and the very craving for the things our tongue liked so well will disappear. After the change to a fruit diet is once established, you will get more pleasure out of your meals than ever before. You will reach a higher degree of existence because you have passed the angel with the flaming sword who guards the gate to paradise.

In conclusion, I want to give you a plain criticism of food value, and that without the help of the high-toned scales of science.

A severe criticism of food values

Meat has no nourishment at all for man. The so-called strength, which we experience after eating is nothing but stimulation. Even the meat-eating animals will die if you feed them on nothing but cooked meat without blood and bones. The same thing happens with an exclusive feeding on eggs, butter or white bread. Even rats will die if you give them nothing but white wheat flour. Those experiments have been made. Nobody can live solely on any one of these so-called good foods. On the other hand, I would bind myself to live on nothing but one kind of fruit for any length of time, and do hard work besides.

Eggs and fats cause the worst impurity of our system. I have found that out with fasters in my sanatorium, who lived before mainly on those foods. I had a millionaire, who was a heavy fat eater who perspired a substance during his fast which was as fat and heavy as melted butter. Cooked and concentrated milk is even worse. It is a mucus former of the first class. Babies may thrive on it in a measure, but how well is proven by the great infantile mortality. All starchy foods are a poor road to grape sugar, which alone can be utilized in the formation of blood. Out of a single fig you will get more nutritive value than out of one pound of bread, rice or potatoes. Milk and starchy foods are the stumbling block for the vegetarian glutton. Dried beans, peas and lentils are causing just as much gout and rheumatism as meat, on account of their high percentage of albumen. Less harmful and more nutritious are all green vegetables, because they contain valuable mineral salts. I use those as a stepping stone to the highest, which is a fruit diet.

Fruits

The adequacy of fruits for human nourishment

is conclusively proven by the fact that the chemical combination is almost the same as mother's milk. Above all, but very little albumen. If mother's milk is sufficient to insure a healthy growth for babies, why should not fruits be an ideal food for the grown-up man? The most decisive test of mother's milk is its sweetness. The most important element of nutrition is not albumen, but organic carbon, so-called "grape-sugar." It has the highest percentage in fruits next to water. Every single fruit contains in ideal combination all the elements needed by the human body. Do you believe for a moment that men can create with chemistry and the use of fire anything superior to that which the Creator has given us from the beginning of time? Anatomically and physiologically man is in close relationship with the apes; this much even the scientists admit. Why, then, should they classify us with the hogs, when they are writing a book on diet? The most overwhelming proof that fruits are the ideal food for man is furnished in the success of an exclusive fruit diet for the cure of chronic diseases. I healed the difficult cases of chronic diseases with fruit diet after everything else failed. I have cured myself from the disease of albuminaria through fasting and a strict diet, and I have reached a degree of health which I did not know before. I have supervised hundreds of such cures with excellent results. If fruits have a healing power and regenerate us, it must follow that they are the best food to keep us in ideal health. Modern life is the *tragedy* of *nutrition*. The curse of civilization is the feverish struggle for the possession of money, so that we might enjoy the so-called privilege of sitting around a well-spread table three times a day; while we do not realize that by doing so we undermine our health and step into an untimely grave.

I hope you will take the conviction with you that you have seen the question of nutrition in a new light of truth. If you come to the decision to turn over a new leaf in your habits of eating, you will gain in proportion to the adherence to these new principles. You will, moreover, serve your country better in this way than in any other. And by following the way I have outlined to you, you give yourself the best treat, because it is an easy and broad way to economic independence as well as to ideal health. Moreover, you people, who live in the most favored fruit country in the world, ought to become the pioneers in this movement to help a suffering humanity to conquer gluttony by a closer adherence to the ideal diet.

Physical Culture

In this dissertation Ehret relates the practice of dietetics and fasting with physical culture to produce the high degree of civilization that prevailed in the age of Old Greece.

A strict interpretation of the word "Civilization" embraces spiritual culture, only, and its scientific meaning can be expressed as the ennobling and perfection of man, in regard to his intellectual, moral and esthetic qualities.

In spite of this, we find that the highest degree of civilization in history (the classic period of the Hellenic Age) combined, or was even based upon a highly developed physical culture.

As a contrast, you may be reminded that the Middle Age is classified in the history of civilization as a kind of spiritual stagnation—thru' its one-sided, nearly exclusive religious development, neglecting the culture of the body, entirely. Nietzsche may be somewhat right when he says: "Christianity has robbed us of the entire classic civilization." Saying this, he surely thought not only on the spitirual—but a great deal on the physical development of the classic Greek and Roman peoples.

The philosophy of Western Civilization is based upon Greek thinking, and the word treasure of all sciences has most of its roots in the Greek and Latin languages.

Esthetics; the science of beauty in the history of European art, especially sculpture and architecture, is based upon the Greek classic example of enduring foundation in principal lines.

There is no better example of the perfect human body than the Apollo and Venus of the classic Hellenic period, and the foot racers of the Marathon exemplify, undoubtedly, a classic example of physical culture.

The Greek of this time were, no doubt, cultivated and developed by physical training and a high standard of Eugenics. The living models of the Gods, reproduced in sculpture by the great artist Phidias—the immortal creator of human beauty.

The gymnasium where unclothed boys and girls, together received their daily physical exercise, as the principle of "classic education" is significant— as regards morals and education.

The "Temple of Aesculap" was mainly, a place for what was known as "The sleep in the Temple." Here all sick people had to go, just as they go to a hospital, today. They were kept sleeping all of the time—which means, fasting.

Regarding the diet of the classic period, we know

very little—but this much is certain, that is: Cooking and eating were not the most important things—as they are in this civilization. I suppose that at the banquets, which are called "Bacchanals," no alcoholic beverages were used. In every artist's conception of this kind of a painting, the grapes are the "significant thing" at the 'Bacchanal" festival.

I believe that a scholar of classic Greek language and civilization, of Greek philosophy, science; Greek art and mythology—and who knows about and believes in physical culture; in fasting and dietetics, at the same time would find and discover this:

The classic age of Greek civilization—which we call the highest in history—was based upon and due to a highly developed body thru' physical culture, fasting, dietetics and Eugenics. As with the Romans—degeneration set in just as soon as gluttony gained ground—as soon as Lucullus and Bacchus became Gods.

The production and development of individual bodily perfection and geniality was the goal of classic Greek civiliztion.

We find another standard of civilization with the old Egyptians—and it is said that their prominent learned men and "High Priests" did not swallow solid foods for decades. They practiced "Fletcherism" some thousand years B. C.

Seen thru' the glasses of dietetics and fasting—hygienic and dietetic rules, you will find that these ideas go, like a red string, thru' the Mosaic legislation—and thru' the stories of physical and spiritual heroes and prophets of the Old and New Testaments.

That physical culture in the classic age of old Greece was combined with fasting and a high standard of dietetics can be proved by the stories of two of the greatest geniuses of history: Pythagoras and Hippocrates.

Pythagoras, an immortal mathematical genius; vegetarian and founder of a high-standing school of philosophy, went to Egypt to learn more about the "secret sciences" of that country. Before he was allowed to enter into the school of the learned, called High Priests at this time, he had to undergo a fast of forty days, under supervision, outside of the city. Believing that this was a test of his will power and energy, he was told this: "Forty days' fast is necessary in order that you may grasp what we will teach you."

Hippocrates, another mathematician, and learned in natural science, is called the "Father of Medicine"—because he was the first to cleanse this "doctrine" from superstition and put it on a scientific basis. However, remarkable as it is—he was an exclusive dietitian. He did not have much knowledge of modern medicine, anatomy and physiology. He knew exactly what disease was, and what was going on in the human body, in case of sickness. His ideas, concept and teachings about how to heal every disease can be characteristically seen and understood by two quotations from his works on dietetics. He says: "The more you feed the sick, the more you harm him." Also—"Your foods shall be your 'remedies,' and your 'remedies' shall be your foods."

His first statement proves clearly that he was an advocate of fasting and restrictive diet, especially in case of acute disease. His second statement (suggestion) embraces perfectly the entire problem of dietetics. It is exactly what I call the "Diet of Healing."

For a clearer understanding, it may be explained as follows: Nature's only and omnipotent "remedy"—fasting—is used in the animal kingdom to heal every disease and wound; showing that there is only one disease. I call it internal impurity—mucus derived from decomposed, un-natural foods. By healing wounds, Nature shows that she can do it better and more perfectly, without food.

In case of disease, Nature, with the instinctive "signal" of non-appetite, strives to say: "You did wrong by eating—stop it—or at least, replace the wrong foods which produced your disease, with good, clean, natural ones. You must do this, if I am to heal you and save you from the consequences of your wrong eating." Or, in the language of the Scriptures: "I am the Lord, thy Physician—my foods, produced by Nature, only, are thy reme- dies—and thou shalt eat only the bread of Heaven—fruits and herbs" (Genesis), meaning greenleaf vegetables.

For thousands of years—since the time of Hippocrates and Moses, the truth has been revealed, but not believed—not understood and followed. Up to the present time, a "radical" diet, such as advocated by Hippocrates, as a diet of healing ("remedies")—and suggested by Moses, as man's natural food, exclusively, has received little credit, even among dietitians.

Why, in our time of regeneration by physical culture, have not fasting and dietetics become the principal and standard "remedy" of natural therapeutics—as it was in the classic age of civilization, as shown above?

As a specialist in fasting and dietetics, with more than twenty years' practice, I submit this slow progress is due to the following facts: First, the modern man—the sick man, especially—is so overloaded with impurities; disease matters, that he cannot endure a long fast. In fact, it would, in many cases, become dangerous. My experience has taught me that shorter fasts, alternating with a cleansing diet, and progressively increased, are much more easy and successful than longer fastings. I call this process a systematical fast. Second: The radical fruit diet; the raw food diet, or, as I call it, the "Mucusless Diet"—(fruits, exclusively; nuts and green-leaf vegetables) stirs up and dissolves too rapidly in the body of the average sick man, with his lowered vitality—so much waste and toxemias that he cannot endure the elimination of same. His condition becomes worse, instead of better, and he and everyone around him attributes it to the lack of solid food; and his faith in natural foods has vanished, forever.

In fact, this is the reason why we have such a confusion in dietetics, today. The amount of nutriment contained in a food is not the decisive point, but, rather, its eliminating qualities determines to what extent it is a "remedy"—according to Hippocrates.

I learned this, mostly, thru' my experience with serious cases of all kinds of disease; and imperfect conditions. The change from wrong, disease-producing foods to right, disease-healing foods, has to be affected slowly, progressively and systematically—according to the condition of the patient.

A diet of healing can never consist of recipes and the prescription of menus for the so-called different kinds of diseases. What I call the "Transition Diet" must be a therapeutic system of eating, for elimination of waste and toxemias (disease matters) selected, adjusted and combined in such a way that the elimination can be controlled. Combined with fasting, we have a system of therapeutics which surpasses any other in existence.

If physical culture of any kind is combined with this system, the elimination can be enforced rapidly. When the body is once clean; free from any waste or poison—when all obstructions are removed from the human machine—then the physical culturist will develop a strength, endurance and a beauty of solid muscular proportion, and, at the same time, enjoy a mental and spiritual progress equalling that of the classic period of the "Hellenic Age."

No doubt our Western civilization is at stake. We drift along in a sort of half-conscious condition—as tho' we were advanced to a high degree of civilization. The average mind thinks that the progress of technic and industry—economic and financial prosperity and success compose civilization. The flight (so-called escape) from healthful physical out-of-door work in the country, into the offices, theaters, restaurants, etc., located in the un-hygienic buildings of large cities, is called progress.

Statistics show that we have the highest record in history in the development of consumption, cancer and syphilis. Whoever has treated chronic cases of this kind, knows the inside story of our so-called progress.

Due to the internal impurity of modern man, his disease (of whatever nature) is of a degree never before attained by any people, in the history of mankind—and this is caused, mainly, thru' his diet of civilization, and to the lack of physical culture.

At the present time we are menaced by an overwhelming culture of psychology; of metaphysics; of spiritualism—of spiritual "manias" of all kinds. It is significant that a well-known teacher of one of these cults had to remind his audience, upon different occasions, during the same lecture: "Yes; you must realize that you have a body." The spiritual confusion; the uncertainty and contradictions found even in science, philosophy and religion, have no analogy in the history of civilization.

The ignorance regarding the most important things in life—the health and perfection of the body—is indescribable. We suffer from a sort of psychic defect; failing to realize how important health is.

We are swimming in an ocean of books, and are brought into such a maelstrom of ideas that no one has a correct conception of the truth—or that health is the most important truth.

The attitude of the human mind towards everything spiritual is so terribly confused that you cannot find two men, today, who can agree on any one idea. This much is certain, however, there are no two truths about the spiritual and physical perfection of the human being. I have shown, thru' "classic examples," that the highest degree of real civilization—of mental and spiritual standards—was reached, and could be reached, only, thru' a most perfect body—thru' a superb, splendid health in every line—developed thru' physical culture, fasting and dietetics.

If the individual will not banish all superstition from his mind, and take care of his body in every respect; he, or she, cannot be saved from disease and imperfection.

Mankind, especially of the Western civilization, must soon take up the culture and care of the body, in the broadest sense—exactly as prevailed in the classic age of Old Greece. The development of this process, alone, will determine whether or not civilization can be saved.

Thus Speaketh the Stomach

Permitting the stomach to speak, Professor Ehret discloses how to find the cause of increased and decreased functional capacity in all parts of the whole system.

The philosopher, Immanuel Kent, and other contemporary thinkers, have ventured to critically investigate the process of thinking, itself. The more modern materialistic school may at least claim the merit of having reminded us that normal thinking requires a normal organ of thought, with well-organized brain convolutions. Materialism placed the carriers of philosophical minds upon earthly soil again. It did not commence its speculations in the background, nor in the abstract, super-sensual and metaphysical—it put the scalpel of its thinking, figuratively and in reality, at the organs of the soul, and opened up a philosophy of life—starting with the material atom, and the cell of living substances. Brain convolutions, and the quality of nerve substance, seemed to become the criterion of a material basis—in order to obtain a "Critique of Pure Reason," without sophistic tendencies, and to grasp the spiritual and physical life—the process of thinking, as perception, logic and judgment. Now, the cell appeared really tangible and visible, as a specifically organized unit of living substance, and, as a co-ordinated carrier of bodily and mental

functions. The anatomy of these micro-organisms
is known; but the quality of their functions, the
causes of their vitality are yet obscure. They forget
that all depends upon the nourishing with live
blood, and that the fundamental lever of all thinking—of thinking, itself—has to be put at the stomach; the center of blood formation—if we want to
solve the mystery of life. One has to go to the
gravity center of the organism—that is, one's stomach—in order to understand; alleviate; remedy the
heaviness; the impediments to one's functions,
known as disease. One has to look into the work-
ings and at the basis of his central organs, if he
wants to find the cause of accelerated and lowered
functional capacity of all parts of the whole system, which are being nourished with blood, by the
stomach.

Jean Jacques Rosseau dictated his writings while in
a recumbent position. Freidrich Von Schiller put
his feet into cold water while writing. Fainting is
often the last stage of a bloodless condition of the
brain, caused thru' a full stomach. Pythagoras had
to fast forty days in order to understand the
wisdom of Egypt; however, not because fasting
causes a bloodless condition of the brain, as is
generally believed, but, because the very opposite
is the case. Far better than recumbent—as with
Rosseau or by cooling the feet—as with Schiller—
does the human brain produce the best thoughts,
the surest perceptions, when thoroughly permeated
with blood. If, by fasting—as with Pythagoras,—the
stomach has been brought to that state of cleanli-

ness whereby perfect digestion of food is assured; there will be no interference in the regular nourishing of the brain with blood—thru' the presence of auto-toxins. One has, eventually to begin at the stomach, with a blood purifying. We must enter upon a higher grade of health—starting from the center of blood formation, in order to obtain a perception of "blood-pure-reason," a priori, that disease in the main is but an unconscious laying of mines in the body, which will be brought to an inflammation and eruption thru' secondary, incident causes, such as a cold, infection, etc. We must eliminate the presence of unevacuated feces, retained thru' sticky mucus in the pockets of the intestines, constantly poisoning, and thereby interfering with proper digestion and blood-building.

Not only all life, but all culture, in the better sense, proceeds from the stomach. But this organ, thru' false nursing by the too-material cult of Bacchus and Lucullus—according to Nietzsche—has become the father of all misery: the secret hot-bed of all disease. Here a latent deposit of moribund matter, consisting of retained waste products, is acting oppressively on the brain, and corrupting the blood, and, in each special case of disease; besides being the direct cause, coming from the obscure, underground stomach cover, it obscures the clinical picture of every symptom of an eliminative nature, for the time being. As can be proved, pounds of the secret, pathological ailment are deposited within the tissues, as a primary cause of disease; as chronic corruption of the blood—coming from the under-ground; the obscure unknown; the mysterious X—in the course of all acute and chronic disease processes.

If, today, in some manner, I may introduce a speaking stomach, this is done for three reasons: First, because this rather antiquated form of expression seems better adapted to impart personal perceptions and concepts. Second, because the functions of an organ; a process of Nature! a force; a will—the sense and purposeful intentions of unconscious partial functions of the human body, when especially personified and given speech, are brought nearer to the general intelligence of the people. Third, because diet and with that, the stomach—the blood formation—are the first things implied in the question: "What and how should we eat and drink, in order to get well, and remain healthy?" Perhaps even science can find some animating thoughts in this idea.

Supported by an extensive material of facts, and by certain experiments upon my own body—such as no one else has made, so far—I will attempt to introduce to you, the stomach—as the gathering place of that pathological material which has generally been called, encumbrance; auto-toxins; morbid disposition, or tendency; without the presence of which, the action of a secondary cause of disease is impossible. I have made experiments to produce a cold; to get malaria infection, etc., with a negative result—after a thorough removal of the first general cause; consisting of the complete encumbrance, thru' the stomach—by fasting and using my own diet. In order to put disease, as an experiment, upon a common basis, I went to the limit of endangering my life. In a state of improved health, I would intentionally eat myself sick, to a certain extent; in order to eat myself surely and radically well, again—for my own satisfaction. To my knowledge, this has never before been attempted. If science does not care about this experimenting of mine—it may continue to look on, smilingly, at what is to follow. I, myself, believe I shall thereby be of service to the sick—to the life efficiency of the human race—to the promotion of the peoples' vigor, and, to all humanity.

And now, let the stomach speak; in the principal role of the "Tragedy of Man's Nutrition."

Thus Speaketh the Stomach:

"Histogenetically, I am, at first, a primitive, intestinal cell; a tiny, hollow bag, with a mouth-opening; this being the ultimate, common, basic form of all true multi-cellular vertebrates—according to Haeckel. In the whole scale of living animal organisms up to and including man, I am located in the center, at the point of gravity. To me—the Stomach—belongs this centrally-located place; for I am the single building spot; the organized working apparatus for raw material, and, at the same time, the master-builder. I get my orders thru' the brain—the chief management—as unconscious instincts, from the world's architect. To me, alone—with my assistant, the blood-stream, belongs, in the main, the material building of the whole body; the formation and

shaping of the organs; their maintenance; and the
supply of repair material. I am the material main
center of growth; replenishing and working the
whole organism. Even the chief management—the
brain—is subject to my food carrier; the blood. I
have always been, and shall remain, the first and
absolute ruler in the cell state of man, and of
animals. To me belongs the center of being and
health; of pain and disease, and of passing away.
Thus I, only, in the first line, can be the source and
supply of remedy—the hot-bed and the death-bed
of disease.

"In the chase after causative factors of disease, I
have been displaced from my dominating position
among the organs, in man's perception—however,
in the scale of so-called pleasures of life and
culture, I have been elevated to the 'Chief God.' In
reality, the millenarian mistreatment of man has
made of me a dark chamber of suicidal table
enjoyment—and pain, my warning voice and de-
fensive force, has been choked in the endless
courses of dimmed kitchens. Man's thinking has
become obscured in the tempo of over-culture of
his abdomen—the conception of health has dissolved in fancy—and the spectre of disease is
haunting him. Also the terror of this phantom; his
suffering and death emanate from me. If I am the
center of life; why should I not, also, be the center
of death.

"Pain, uneasiness in general—and in particular
parts—are my signals to: 'Stop! too much unnecessary eating!' These are alarm dispatches, and indi-

cate functional disturbances in the vascular system, as a reaction on me—which I ingeniously support by loss of appetite. They answer me by strangling my voice, thru' more eating. My voice works as a danger signal, causing pain—because, thru' over-eating and drinking, the pressure and density of blood are increased by me, instead of being diminished. In the state of disease and elimination, the blood stream carries the dissolved auto-toxins from me to the kidneys; this goes on painlessly, with relaxed tissues, only while fasting—which acts as a relief. Pain is merely my cry of distress; an expression of my disturbed healing work, which I can perform, thoroughly, only when I am empty and fasting. In fact and truth, my pain signals are good and life-promoting; thought and action-provoking to thinking people. They should be the refining fire; the upward move for the overcoming of suffering and disease—the fore-runner of a new dawn of life. (These ideas may serve as a contribution to the Philosophy of Suffering; or Revelation of all values.)

"I, the Stomach, am the primary ruler over life and death; from the first primitive intestinal cell, to the passing away of the last creature. My rule over living beings is self-evident—as I am the first deciding court of remedy; of repair; of restoration of the functional and organic disturbances called disease. Unceasingly, with the help of the organs of elimination and protection, I am secretely at work; to regulate the well-being of man with Edenic reserve forces. Especially in advanced years, I maintain a secret process of life-protecting and life-sustaining

purpose; in the most subtle form. Under continued
inflow of unassimilable matter, of so-called food
culture, and, especially, during the stoppage of my
drainage canal, I am unable to maintain the balance. I become flabby, from the eliminating work,
and so does the whole tissue and blood system of
my surroundings, and, of the entire body. I can
neither digest the inflow, nor overcome it by
secretion. I have to deposit matter for more tran-
quil times and store it up in the tissues. Abnormal
distension of my cavity and of the whole body, is
called 'vigorous health'—which must be registered
by a pathological condition.

"My 'striking'; and the possibility of eliminating
the morbid matter of putrescent refuse, consists in
absolute emptiness and sobriety of fasting—and on
an instinctive animal command of the 'world regis-
seur.' My intention is good—a regulating of the
health and running-activity—a sort of self-de-
fense—an aid from the underground. Instead of
properly defending yourselves against all enemies
and dangers of life, you have throttled my life and
healing activities—my digestive power and my eating capacity. My glands, my walls, the tissues of
my surroundings, and, especially, my ten meter
long canal, are permeated, infected, soiled, in
proportion to my chronic abuse, thru' modern
eating. At the basis of my tissues, especially those
of my surroundings. I have to deposit the residue,
which, in the course of all disease, remains unknown to you; as the primary cause—because, only
while I am empty and fasting, can I attack it;

devour it; work it off; burn it up; and healingly eliminate it thru' the blood stream.

"Instead of being a fountain of wholesome life—the source of purest blood and health—I have become the secret underground chamber; the breeding place of all suffering, and the father of all misery.

"Thus I take up my 'song of lamentation,' as the most temperate representative of the present time. 'He that hath ears to hear, let him hear.' Already, in the womb of the mother—out of care for a new human life—I induce disgust for unnatural 'cultured' eating—to retain the purity of the blood, and to conform with the instinct for primitive nutrition, thru' fruit. However, I am fed double rations—and they wonder why the birth takes place with pain, and danger to life for mother and child. I am given food poor in minerals, especially in lime—such as flesh, boiled, decalcified milk; while I long for the lime salts of fruits—since I have to build up a new bony frame for the embryo. I catch up every milligram of lime salts, even at the expense of the mother's teeth; in order to give it to the child, in formation. Hysteria, and caries of the teeth of the pregnant, is how they diagnose my care for a new human life. I am unable to build good mother's milk substance; since I am lacking in fruit sugar; its main ingredient—altho' I am flooded with cow's milk. I am also kept well supplied with this during the nursing period of the young one—also with the entire list of imaginable slime preparations. I cannot overcome the cheesy, putrescent refuse, and the slimy condition reaches from the throat to the pasted and clogged-up outlet. My interior is stuffed with boiled, pallid, curdled and decalcified milk, and its germ-producing condition threatens to strangle the windpipe of the little one. I am laboring with obstructions, impediments and friction; in fever heat. By forceful, downward pressure, I try to make room, but my good intentions are frustrated thru' constipating drugs. Now I have the emergency vents of the skin open to throw off waste and impurities, that slide into the blood stream.

"Measles, scarlet fever, eruptions—they call my last efforts to throw off the morbid; the useless; the disease germs. If, in spite of all, the young citizen succeeds in getting on his legs; he at once searches for sweets and fruits; to which I urge him, with Edenic instinct. The live elements of fruit sugar give me a chance for a radical discharge of the putrescent mucus masses that have accumulated into a dangerous breeding field, within myself— with a stench reminding one of carrion and death. I discharge the first layer of my own depository of disease, and that of the intestines, as a warning to reform; and as a sign of my good intentions as to 'life insurance.' This is called loose stool: scientifically known as diarrhea and colitis; and is stopped by opium. Since my evacuations originate from putrid, curdled milk, they are of greenish color. With adults, especially with heavy meat eaters, they are blackish. In extreme cases of my defense work, downward, as well as upward, they speak more learnedly of Cholera morbus. If, thru' climatic heat, the danger of fermentation is still greater, and my provisional eruptions more intense; then my attempts at cleansing from slime and bacillus soil is called Cholera Asiatica—with which one usually smothers in his own morass; because he counteracts my eliminative efforts. When attempting to gradually accustom my youthful purity to meat, liquors, etc., I respond, in the child, with squeamishness, and, in my juvenile elasticity, I try to eject the loathsome, unnatural stuff, thru' energetic contractions. This is called 'colic'; and with the aid of the rod, they force the reactive youngster to weaken my original power, thru' so-called strengthening food.

"At the age of puberty, I start my special effort at cleansing, with the woman—in the organ of gestation—to take place regularly each month, before the period of possible conception; with the sole purpose of cleansing before fecundation. This phenomenon is the health-regulating process of disease; and is lessened both as to quantity and frequency, in proportion to the general efforts at cleansing; commencing with me. It becomes superfluous and disappears entirely, with perfect health—if I am fed exclusively on pure and unmixed food, with fruit, alone. (For proof; we refer to the lives of many saints.) I am likewise interested in the formation of pure blood in the young man, since the quality of his blood is not only of importance to him; but to his whole future generation. The sins of the ancestors, and the germs of immortality are in the atmosphere of today, but,

with me, nobody has dared to find them. The
entire list of sexuo-pathological symptoms may be
pretty closely produced thru' a one-sided, extreme
increase in feeding on 'food of the beasts of prey.'
Do you know that you can kill a man by feeding
him exclusively on flesh—the much-lauded main
food of the century?

"With the Stomach, also, 'talking amounts to
silver,' while silence is often worth gold; especially,
when one's stomach could speak whole volumes
about the foolishness of people, but without avail.
To the asthmatic I give timely warnings of my
uneasiness due to lack of oxygen in the digestion. I
control the elimination and subsequent emaciation
in these types, especially. 'Tuberculosis has a certain healing tendency,' said Prof. Virchow, the
great pathologist. This disease also originates with
me—in the underground—destroying the air-organ,
when I cannot get any more air, on account of
wrong eating. To overcome the highest degree of
blood corruption and the breakdown of the entire
cell-state—as in the case of tuberculosis and cancer,
my blood stream seeks to get a crater-like eruption
spot; and an emergency vent, as it were, to throw
off the products of decay, viz: slime and pus. At
the very beginning, before the process of eruption,
I ulcerate the surroundings; while depositing, germinating and re-building—for the filth is of especially
putrefactive origin—resulting from excessive consumption of flesh and eggs. In most cases of this
kind, I—the builder of man's body—am able to be
of material help—and, if they attempt to assist me
with their 'best diet,' they only make things worse.

"Do they not even try to regulate the heart beat, thru' means which I have to take? Then why should not I also be the 'father of tortured hearts,' when I, thru' high pressure, must poison and corrupt the blood which is banked up in the chambers of this valve; congesting the air pump (the lungs) where gas—oxygen, is lacking? Not only must I, as the breeding and blood forming place —produce germs of putrefaction—in the field of underground encumbrance, but, by force of emergency the pathological matter even forms into crystallized, stony condensations; obstructing the blood stream in narrow passage-ways (as in the case of rheumatism) or being deposited as stones in the gall bladder, or in the notches of the intestines.

"The resisting bulwark and greatest counter-force; the greatest impediment—which makes it possible to prevent this germ depositary of all diseases—is chronic constipation; the obstruction of the end of my drainage pipe; the rectum. Of the upper portion of my auxiliary organ—the intestinal canal— only one part need be mentioned here. In sheer blindness, they mistook the appendix for a 'blind'—superfluous and even impending structure, which, however, was to assist in the lubrication and smoothening of the chyle; thru' its secretion—like the oiler of a machine. Naturally, a machine will run for a time with a clogged-up oiler; or without same—but only until it becomes burning hot."

"Still greater than within myself and my surroundings, is the accumulation of filth at the outlet of

the drainage pipe. Thru' decades of damming up,
there has gathered a mire-like mass beyond descrip-
tion. The deep folds conceal heaps of slime and
fecal matter, in stony formation of many years'
standing. This ulcerating and fermenting depository
of putrefying refuse of the process of disintegration of one's own tissues, is, in conjunction with
myself, a first-class hot bed and breeding place of
all diseases. Here is the dark, secret, underground
reservoir of the dietary mire, which is poisoning
the blood-stream from childhood on, and, like an
obscure subterranean spring, is feeding all painful
disease symptoms. There we find the deeper causes
of apoplexy, neurasthenia, typhus, head troubles,
kidney and liver infections—and of the varied list
of 'specialties' invented by the 'medical brain.' I,
the principal organ of digestion, like all other parts;
especially the injured tissues of blood vessels con-
gested by a cold—continuously receive from this
reservoir deadly excremental gases and substances,
thru' the circulation—and I even stir up this partially dead chamber, within a living body, because I
must, naturally, expel my contents thereinto.

"Germs of decayed and live parasites, broods of
vermin of various species, live and thrive on the
refuse of flesh and starch in the alimentary canals
of un-numbered people; displaying a good appetite,
and a voracity for the favored food of these pests.
Fruit acids would kill them—but my interior walls,
and my reflecting image, the taste-organ (tongue),
are so charged with slime and so pasty that I
cannot make known my primitive instinct for fruit.
Air; water; sunshine; fruit sugar; fruit acids—and

the building stones of organized substances containing albumen in the maximum of one-half per cent, were, originally, and still are the sole and natural components of my helio-electric formation of blood—with radio-active force from sweet scents and odors of fruits; 'the bread of Heaven.'

"I was, originally, tuned to a mono-diet consisting of a varied selection from the fruits in season, differing in the degree of their water value, and in accordance with the position of the sun and the average temperature of the respective zones. Out of these, I produced force and warmth; bone and muscle, for Edenic man, healthy and free from disease germs—just as today with the frugivorous apes; or with quadrupeds, on grass and water, in twenty degrees below zero.

"I can ward off and expel the much-accused poisons of modern civilization, such as alcohol, coffee, tobacco, etc., in much less time than I can throw off the ballast of 'cultured' eating, which has become the custom. The continuous overloading therewith, in disgusting mixtures, and without necessity, threatens to choke and drown me, and my life functions. Within me, on a base of soups, beer and wine, there is constantly swimming a varied and heterogeneous mixture of unchewed and useless substances, which are already largely decomposed—out of which I am supposed to turn out the live ingredients of the blood.

"The first thing to do would be to value all eatables accordingly—so that none of the necessary secretions and excretions would adhere to me, or to any part of the digestive apparatus; encumbering and obstructing everything with pasty slime—and to liberate me, first of all, from all slime permeating my structure—thru' the use of dissolving foods, especially fruits, salads and vegetables.

"To be, or not to be, healthy or sick—the life and death of man and humanity lies within my power. I am the ultimate smithery and destiny to all men. According to natural law and purpose, I am the hammer which can fashion out of blood and iron, men with vigorous, indestructible health. To be sure, it takes live blood made out of the meat of grapes, oranges and such fruits, full of organic iron—instead of dead animals, with disintegrated and devitalized albuminous matter. I seem only to have become the anvil on which they think to weld dead matter into live substance. My silent, Edenic harmony has been turned into dull growling. I already spit sparks of fire which will consume him who means to throttle me. His downfall is my paternal blood on the stage of life, in the Tragedy of Man's Nutrition.

"Thus sounds my lamentation: I, and my auxiliary organs, have been proven, in the zoological order of evolution—with 'moral glory'—to be the organs of beasts of prey—and, in the biological order, from a dietetic and physiological standpoint, we have been out on a level with the swine—in order to justify the modern diet. All species and varieties I must digest; from the mollusks of the sea to the ruminants of the field, and the birds of the air—and I have, apparently, adapted myself to their form of nutrition. Man has lost the appetite for fruits—the primary diet of the human stomach—and the faith in their live power (according to Dr. Bircher-Benner.) The genealogy of man may be traced back to the ape family, thru' a queer branching off—but, in the present condition of my auxiliary organs, the teeth and intestines; and of myself, my brotherly similarity to the frugivorous ape, in regard to diet, has been denied.

"Man was formerly content to be satisfied with a few fruits of the forest, in order to procreate god-like, Edenic human beings, as the predecessors of the hunter, with spear and fire. I am still existing on this pre-historic reserve fund of force; while dissipating my capital fund in the digestion of luxuries. My present silence—while being fed on milk, eggs, flesh, cereals and pulses, liquors, and the entire modern artificial diet, speaks volumes. My glands, and the introductory structures of my tract are clogged with a slimy, sticky mucus, which has ruined them. The sensory and defensory nerves are benumbed. With the patience of a giant, I endure the ten-fold measure and carrion-like quality of the meals, lauded as good and strengthening—while they are the very opposite—weakening and inducing incapacity to react against unassimilable matter. In fact, I operate under great difficulties, and 'keep the machine going' with the most necessary water and air. They call my silence under the strain of desperate effort—and the mute patience of a giant—'good digestion.' While the organic wheel is jarring, heaving and groaning, and the pipes threaten to burst.

"Grapes, cherries, apples, all sweet and sour fruits I easily digest and turn into pure blood, thru' my Edenic capacities—only when I have thereby eliminated and ejected the last remnant of refuse matter, accumulated during a lifetime. If you again extend the hand of reconciliation, for the 'bread of Heaven,' and you want to eat yourself well, then I commence the most ingenious mining work, with the new blood from the sun kitchen. With it, I work thru' the whole body, stirring up the old, latent disease germs, and especially, the new-symptom fields. I begin the healing and transmutation of the entire man. The most radical cleansing of myself, and of my surroundings—particularly of my drainage system, which is full of retained refuse matter, furnishing the real reduction of the entire encumbrance—and manifesting itself in an alarming emaciation. However, I can only commence my constructive, nourishing work with fruits, after all worn-out building material of my mansion has been removed. I can then, only, become again the fountain of health; the wall of life; the inexhaustible source of vigor and pleasure—altho', hereditarily, since Adam; thru' milleniums, and, individually, for decades, I have been the father of misery, and the germinating center of all diseases and afflictions."

The Definite Cure of Chronic Constipation

After four years of exacting study and dangerous experimenting on his own body Ehret discovered the following: Disease is Nature's effort to rid the body of disease matters and to eliminate waste from the system. Instinctively the voice of Nature comes to man as it does to animals, "Don't eat — rest — be quiet!"

Chronic constipation is the worst and most common crime against life and mankind — a crime unconsciously committed, and one whose full enormity is not yet fully realized. It stands accused of being one of the principal causative factors of all physical and mental diseases. I know as a fact, from my practical experience with thousands of chronically diseased, that the life of man, and the extent of his mental and spiritual capabilities are largely influenced by the condition of the alimentary tract. It is certainly very important that the brain and nerves of man are supplied with pure blood, and are not dependent on blood, polluted with impurities, arising from an unclean alimentary canal. "Unclean" is too mild a word, when we are dealing with the worst kind of a filthy condition.

It is a fact that man, the product of the present "civilized" society of this much vaunted "advanced" twentieth century, is born in filth, because his mother, during pregnancy, is almost invariably suffering from constipation. And I say further, that while in this state, she usually eats two to three times as much as is necessary. This causes the so-called normal, more or less healthy man, to be somewhat encumbered from infancy. And to a much greater extent, is the constipated one — who is loaded with such a mass of internal filth, that it can only be called "indescribable." His alimentary tract, reaching up from the mouth of the anus to his throat, is filled with a morbid mucus — undigested, decayed and retained food-substances, all of which are in a state of fermentation and putrefaction. His intestines have never had a perfect cleansing during his entire life. At the conclusion of each discharge, the anus must be artificially cleansed, which shows that the internal walls of the intestines must also retain, after each passage, quantities of this same filth.

A physician of Berlin, whose life work was the performing of autopsies, stated that 60 per cent of all the corpses contained in the alimentary canal various foreign matter — worms and petrified feces — and he further stated that in nearly all cases the walls of the intestines and colon were lined with a crust of hardened feces, making it evident that these organs had degenerated to a state of utter inefficiency. Progressive American physicians are rapidly awakening to the fact that retained fecal matter is one of the chief causes of disease. Autopsies are constantly revealing indescribable filthy astounding conditions. One physician publishes the following:

"I have found a prototype of the cause of all diseases of the human body, the foundation of premature old age and death. Surprising as it may seem, out of two hundred and eighty-four cases of autopsy held, but twenty-eight colons were found to be free from hardened feces and in a normal and healthy state. The others, as described above, were to a more or less extent incrusted with hardened, rotten, rejected food material. Many were distended to twice their natural size throughout their whole length with a small hole through the center and almost universally these last cases mentioned had regular bowel evacuations daily. Some of them contained large worms from four to six inches in length.

"My experience from day to day developed startling discoveries in the form of worms and nests of eggs, that we daily get from patients, accompanied by blood and pus. As I stood looking at the colon and reservoir of death, I expressed myself in wonder that anyone can live a week, much less for years, with such a cesspool of death and contagion always with him. The absorption of the deadly poison back into the circulation cannot help but cause all the contagious diseases. The recent treatment of hemorrhage of the bowels in typhoid fever has shown it to be caused by maggots and worms eating into the sensitive membrane and tapping a vein or artery. In fact, my experience during the past ten years has proven, by the rapid recovery of all diseases after the colon was cleansed, that in the colon itself lies the basic cause of almost all human ailments."

That this revolting and indescribable condition arises from the almost universal ignorance of right selection of food, reveals why the "Mucusless Diet Healing System" is such an important discovery and development for the regeneration of mankind.

On the outside, the man of today is carefully groomed, perhaps unnecessarily and over carefully clean; while inside he is dirtier than the dirtiest animal — whose anus is as clean as its mouth, provided said animal has not been "domesticated" by "civilized" man.

Long ago Natural Therapy proved, that in every disease there is a constitutional encumbrance of foreign matter a clogging-up of the system. That statement of fact is not sufficiently explicit. The encumbering matters, foreign to the body, and of no use to the system, consist of masses of accumulated feces, undigested food, morbid mucus, and retained superflous water, all in a state of fermentation and decomposition. Truly, chronically constipated man constantly carries in his intestines a veritable cesspool, by which the blood stream is continually polluted and poisoned, a fact which only a skilled observer can at once detect by facial diagnosis. Official medical science and the inexpert layman do not suspect "constipation" when the individual consumes from three to five meals a day, while he is having one so-called, good bowel movement. Man imagines that his "comfortable fatted" body is a sign of health; at the same time he is as much in fear of a cold wind and "germs" as he is of the devil. When such a "well-fed" man who is usually constipated, takes a fast or is put on a "mucus-less diet" — as I have advised hundreds as their last resort — he will discharge masses of putrescent filth, fetid urine loaded with mucus, salt, uric acid, fat, drugs, albumen and pus, according to his disease.

The most surprising effect of these treatments is the immense quantity of the discharged feces and the fetid exhalation from both the mouth and skin. But the most important "discharge" is the elimination through the circulation into the urine. The urine of everybody will then show a sediment of mucus as soon as he fasts a little or reduces the quantity of his food, or makes a change toward natural, mucusless foods. Doctors call it "disease" and it is in fact a self-cleansing process of the body. This self-elimination through the circulation is the body's most wonderful healing work of every disease. To control this process by food and food quantities is the only true, natural and most perfect therapeutic art of healing and is in no other "treatment" so successfully accomplished as in the "Mucusless Diet Healing System."

This elimination — especially that of the sick man after a long period of misery, suffering and unsuccessful medical treatment — is man's "greatest event." He now realizes what he had never thought of — and what only a few physicians in the world have ever understood as I did, through thousands of cases — that mostly all civilized men are walking, living cesspools, due to chronic constipation.

All his former unsuccessful treatments now appear to him in a tragic-comical light. He now knows exactly where the source of his suffering is to be found, no matter what the name of the disease may be. He now understands that he was wrongly and ignorantly treated by the doctors who "suppressed the disease," without eliminating the filth, which was retained in his entire system, especially in his alimentary canal, since childhood, and which condition constituted the principal causative factor of the disease.

The Effect of Laxatives

I do not believe that either physicians or laymen really know or understand how and why the body performs the laxative effect of these different remedies. Official medical science knows very little about the "why" of the drugs. Their application is based upon the experience only that each one has "a special effect."

All laxatives contain more or less poisons, that is, substances which would become dangerous if they were to enter the circulation in a concentrated form. The protective instinct of the body reacts instantly by a greater water supply into the stomach from the blood in order to dissolve and weaken the dangerous substance; the intestines are stimulated for increased and quickened activity, and so the "solution" is discharged, only taking parts of the feces along. This is the physiological explanation, and you can see that the effect is an abnormal stimulation of vitality in general, and of the intestinal nerves in particular. It is an open secret that all laxatives finally fail, because the constant overloaded intestines are being over-stimulated by the laxatives and thereby slowly paralyzed. To continually increase the laxatives year after year, instead of changing the diet, means SUICIDE — slow, but sure.

The Real and Deeper Cause of Constipation

Constipation itself is a disease, and a really "severe" one, at that, because in severe cases it burdens the system with a heavy load of filth, sometimes weighing as much as ten pounds or more. Disease as such is an abnormal, unnatural condition; even "orthodox" physicians agree on that. We should expire slowly and painlessly, when vitality is exhausted, had we not lived with disease and suffering. That cases of "natural death" are getting more infrequent nowadays is further proof of the depths we have sunken into in the "swamps of civilization."

Constipation — this most common disease — has not decreased or improved in spite of thousands of remedies for sale on the market, and in spite of so-called medical science; simply, because the "diet of civilization" is unnatural. The human intestines are not organized at all for this unnatural food to either digest it perfectly, or to expel the unused residue.

Very little is known about foods that are constipating, and those of the opposite kind. What I wrote and proved in my book, "Rational Fasting and Regeneration Diet," regarding the fundamental causative factors of all diseases, constitutes the deepest insight known into the nature of chronic constipation.

Don't you know that bookbinder's paste is made of fine white flour, rice or potatoes? That glue is made from flesh, gristle and bones? Don't you know how sticky these substances are? Don't you know that skimmed milk, buttermilk and cream are the best ingredients used to furnish sticky base for colors for painting? That the white of eggs will stick paper or cloths so perfectly that it resists dissolution in water? Every housewife and cook knows how oils and fats stick to the sides of a pan. At least 90 per cent of the "diet of civilization" contains these sticky foods and man stuffs himself daily with awful mixtures of them. Thus the digestive tract is not only clogged up through constipation, but literally glued together with sticky mucus and feces.

Herewith the "mystery" of chronic constipation is unveiled and the story told of the fundamental causative factor of all diseases. Disease is but internal uncleanliness — this simply states a true but woeful fact. Fruits, green leaf and starchless vegetables do not contain these pasty, gluey mucus substances and are natural foods — yet little credit has been given them by doctors or laymen. I will lift the veil and show why they fail to understand. Fruit acids and mineral rich vegetables saps — dissolves the pasty mucus encumbrance and fruit sugar causes and develops their fermentation and forms gases. This so greatly feared fermentation of the inside filth is another necessary stirring up "process" to prepare them for elimination. Acid and fermented starch and glue lose their sticky ability as soon as they ferment. If an average meat eater or a child fed mostly on starchy foods accidentally eats too freely of good, sweet fruits, a "revolution" in the alimentary canal, with diarrhea usually sets in (extreme cases are called dysentery cholera), and fever is caused through the increased fermentation.

In severe cases, if a doctor stops the diarrhea and feeds, as is usually the procedure, the patient dies, because nature was kept from accomplishing the cleansing process, and the partly dissolved poisons remain in the system, causing death.

The patient literally suffocates in his own mire of filth, accumulated during his life from wrong food material and over-eating. If he does not die, his case ordinarily becomes chronic, which means: Nature is continually trying to expel poisonous mucus and gases, in spite of all obstructions and counteracting remedies. The constipation merely aggravates the process. Instead of eating less and then only loosening foods, the chronic patient stuffs himself more and more with wrong foods, becomes fatter every day and even takes pleasure in his increased weight. In fact, this over-weight, called health by the misguided ones, is mostly accumulated feces — water — and various kinds of filth. In most cases of tuberculosis, these conditions are typical. Five to six meals a day and one bowel movement or even less — no wonder he takes on weight, looks "full of vigor" — but can never be cured.

Nourishing and Curing Laxatives

No advanced physician will deny the relation between any disease and constipation. But today people are far away from Nature and the truth, and they are kept more and more in darkness — when taken sick they do just the opposite of what they should do. The slightest indisposition, a little headache or cold, which is the result of insufficient bowel movement, is treated with more, and so-called better eating — in spite of a decreased appetite. This is the main reason why Influenza, the "Flu," became a fatal disease. Formerly "Flu" was as easy to cure as the harmless "Grippe" — a self-cleansing process of the body, mostly prevalent in springtime. Knowing nothing of "scientific medicine," germs, etc., the patient instinctively followed his lack of appetite, took a mild laxative and very rapidly recovered; usually he felt much better after than before the "healing" disease. Today, he is falsely taught that a germ is responsible — and not his dangerous unhygienic habits. He eats too much, which is against the law of Nature, instead of fasting, the way every ailing animal cures itself. But the amount of internal impurities and auto-toxins of man exceed those of any diseased animal. A long fast, therefore, would kill the majority of sick men; however, they would not die by starvation, but would become suffocated from their own poisonous filth. As an authority in fasting I know full well the reason why a fast is so feared by most people, and that it has been misapplied by laymen. It is a crime to advise a constipated patient to fast until his tongue is clean, before removing the "deposits of poisons" from his intestines. I could only succeed in curing very old, severe cases of chronic constipation by relatively long fasts. Man, in regard to health, is more degenerated than any kind of animal. He lost his reason, so to say, about matters of which he thinks the animal has none at all. Yet! his intelligence places him far above the animal and enables him to assist Nature to overcome obstructions and difficulties that could become dangerous. That is the philosophical sense of the Art of Natural Healing.

Therefore, if you want to cure chronic constipation perfectly and without any harm, you must change your diet, and instead of using foods which produce disease and constipation, eat really nourishing foods which loosen up, dissolve and cure. But people are ignorant regarding this truth just as they are about fasting, and they try to do things without previous experience or knowledge, and failure is usually the result. What I call "Mucusless Diet" consists of fresh, ripe fruits and starchless vegetables, for they are the ideal foods, and the fundamental remedies for all diseases. Of course, the application must be intelligently advised by personal knowledge which can be received through the study of my book, the "Mucusless Diet Healing System."

It is an "eating-your-way-to-health" treatment, and consequently the most reasonable method of curing, because wrong eating is the causative factor in all diseases.

These mucusless, nourishing and "laxative," that is dissolving, foods form new blood; the best blood that has ever run through your veins — and at once start the so-called constitutional cure of the body. The circulation of the new blood, permeating every part of the system, dissolves and eliminates the morbid mucus, which is clogging up the entire human organism; it especially loosens the deep-seated impurities in the intestines and renovates the whole system. This, then is the great enlightening fact — why constipation not only can be perfectly cured, but why the "Mucusless Diet" cures when all other treatments have failed.

In severe cases of chronic constipation it is advisable, in the beginning, to use as a help, a harmless laxative, to remove the solid obstructions of feces in the intestines; in other words, to eject the worst filth out of a clogged-up pipe system. Enemas consisting of clear, warm water are also a good help in the beginning.

Among numerous laxatives on the market those of vegetable origin are the least harmful. After many years of experience, I have prepared a "special mixture" of this kind. It has the advantage of removing the old, solid feces, obstructions and mucus, from the intestines, without causing the usual diarrhea and constipation as an after effect. It is to be used in the beginning only as an aid, and will not have to be used continually.

As soon as the intestines are cleansed from the retained masses of feces and other obstructions and the mucusless or mucus lean diet is taken up, you will realize the truth of the previously stated facts. You will then perceive with both your eyes and with your nose that I have not exaggerated. And you will become convinced that the state of obstruction was not only localized in your intestines, but that all passages of your entire system were obstructed and constipated with mucus, from your head to your toes.

You will then experience the formerly unbelievable fact — that any kind of disease — even those considered incurable by all doctors — under my treatment soon begin to improve and are finally cured, if a cure is at all possible, simply because the source of poisoning of the system — the chronic constipa-

tion — is eliminated. Then the new blood, derived
from natural food, circulates "unpoisoned" through
the entire system and dissolves and eliminates
every local symptom, even in the most deep-seated
cases; and it removes the impurities of the entire system, which were mainly supplied from
the deposits of poisons and morbid mucus in
the intestines, which condition is called Chronic
Constipation.

Conclusion

"Life is a tragedy of nutrition" is a statement I
made many years ago. Everyone knows we dig our
graves with our teeth, but the saddest of all is the
present-day superstition of 99 percent of the people — the most highly educated and the ignorant — the healthy as well as sick — the rich and
the poor — that we must eat more concentrated
food when weak or sick. Concentrated food, high
protein and starchy foods are the most constipating which, as shown in this booklet, accumulate in
the form of waste in the alimentary canal. The so-
called "good stool" daily is in reality constipation
and you may now see that constipation is the main
source of every disease and that the average person suffering from constipation can only be healed
perfectly by a diet, free from STICKY — GLUEY —
PASTY properties and that is a MUCUSLESS
DIET.

You may improve your elimination temporarily
through laxative remedies — special physical ex-

ercises — vibration, massages and various other methods, but you cannot clean out the old obstructions from the alimentary canal and regenerate and cleanse the whole system as long as you eat the same mucus and toxic-forming foods which have caused and continue causing your constipation and all other ailments of the human body.

The Exact Diagnosis of Your Disease and "The Magic Mirror"

The "mirror" on your tongue's surface reveals the amount of encumbrance that has been clogging up your system since childhood, through wrong, mucus-forming foods — states Professor Arnold Ehret in this article that supports his theory with simple logic.

Since man degenerated through civilization, he no longer knows what to do when he becomes sick. Disease remains the same mystery to modern medical science as it was to the "Medicine Man" of thousands of years ago — the main difference being that the "germ" theory has replaced the "Demon"; and that mysterious, outside power still remains — to harm you and destroy your life.

Disease is a mystery to you as well as to every doctor who has not as yet had a look into the "magic mirror" which I am about to explain. Naturopathy deserves full credit for having proven that disease is within you — a foreign matter which has weight — and which must be eliminated.

If you want to become your own physician, or, if you are a Drugless Healer and want more success, you must learn the truth and know what disease is. You cannot heal yourself, or other people, without an exact diagnosis which will give you a clear idea of true conditions. This infallible truth can be learned only from the book of Nature — that is: Through a test on your own body — or the "magic mirror," as I have designated it.

The sufferer from any kind of disease — or any person, whether sick, or not — who will go through this healing process of fasting and mucusless diet, will eliminate mucus — thereby demonstrating that the basic cause of all latent diseases of man is a clogged-up tissue system of un-eliminated, un-used and un-digested food substances.

Through the "magic mirror" a true and unfailing diagnosis of your disease is furnished, as never before.

"The Magic Mirror"

1. Proof that your personal, individual symptom, sore, or sensation, according to what your disease is named, is nothing more than an extraordinary local accumulation of waste.

2. The coated tongue is evidence of a constitutional encumbrance throughout the entire system, which obstructs and congests the circulation by dissolved mucus, and this mucus even appears in the urine.

3. The presence of unevacuated feces, retained through sticky mucus in the pockets of the intestines, constantly poisoning, and thereby interfering with proper digestion and blood-building.

You will become convinced of this fact — of this diagnosis of your disease — by another surprise in store for you; if you will clean your intestines both before and after the test, with a harmless herb-vegetable compound.

To look inside your body — clearer and far better than can be done by doctors with their expensive X-ray apparatus — and learn the cause of your disease, or even discover some hitherto unknown physical imperfection or mental condition, try this:

Fast one or two days, or eat only fruits for two or three days, and you will notice that your tongue will become heavily coated. When this happens to the acutely sick, the doctor's conclusion is — "indigestion." The tongue is the mirror not only of the stomach, but of the entire membrane system, as well. The fact that this heavy coating returns, even if removed once or twice a day, is an indication of the amount of filth, mucus and other poisons accumulated in the tissues of your entire system, now being eliminated on the inside surface of the stomach, intestines and every cavity of your body.

As soon as you have fasted, decrease the quantity of your food — or eat natural, thereby cleansing, mucusless foods (fruits and starchless vegetables) affording the body an opportunity to loosen and eliminate mucus, which is, in fact, the healing process.

This "mirror" on the tongue's surface reveals to the observer the amount of encumbrance that has been clogging up the system since childhood — through wrong mucus-forming foods. After observing the urine during this test, you will note the elimination of quantities of mucus in same.

The actual amount of filth and waste, which is the "mysterious" cause of your "trouble," is unbelievable.

Disease — every disease — is, first: A special, local constipation of the circulation; tissues; pipe system. The manifestation of symptoms, or, of the different symptoms. If painful and inflamed, it is from over-pressure — heat from friction and congestion.

Second: Disease — every disease —is constitutional constipation. The entire human pipe system, especially the microscopically small capillaries are "chronically" constipated, from the wrong food of civilization.

White blood corpuscles are waste — and there is no man in Western civilization who has mucus-free blood and mucus-free blood vessels. It is like the soot in a stove-pipe which has never been cleaned; in fact, worse — because the waste from protein and starchy foods is STICKY.

The characteristics of tissue construction, especially of the important internal organs, such as the lungs, kidneys, all glands, etc., are very much similar to those of a sponge. Imagine a sponge soaked in paste or glue!

Naturopathy must, more and more, cleanse its science from medical superstitions — wrongly called "scientific diagnosis." Nature, alone, is the teacher of a standard science of truth. She heals by one thing — fasting — every disease that it is possible to heal. This, alone, is proof that Nature recognizes but one disease, and that in every body the largest factor is always, waste, foreign matter and mucus (besides uric acid and other toxemias, and, very often, pus — if tissues are decomposed).

In order to realize how terribly clogged up the human body is, one must have seen thousands of fasters — as I have. The almost inconceivable fact is: How can such quantities of waste be stored up in the body? Have you ever stopped to realize the masses of phlegm you expel during a cold? Just as takes place in your head — your bronchial tubes, lungs, stomach, kidneys, bladder, etc., have the same appearance. All are in the same condition. And the spongy organ known as the tongue shows on its surface how every other part of your body appears.

Medicine has devised a "special science" of laboratory tests, urinal diagnosis and blood tests.
More than fifty years ago, the most prominent pio-

neers of Naturopathy said: "Every disease is foreign matter — waste." I said, twenty years ago, and repeat it again and again, that most of these foreign matters is waste from wrong foods, decomposed — to be seen when it leaves the body as mucus. Meat decomposes into pus.

The light of truth dawned upon me after I had fasted, against the will of the Naturopath from whom I was taking treatments for Bright's disease. When the test-tube filled up with albumen, I read his thoughts in his facial expression. But it proved to me that whatever Nature expels — eliminates — is waste; whether it be albumen, sugar, mineral salts or uric acid. This occurred more than twenty-four years ago, but this Nature-doctor (a former M.D.) still believes in the replacement of albumen by high protein foods.

The medical diagnosis of Bright's Disease, when the chemical test of urine shows a high percentage of albumen, is as misleading as others. The elimination of albumen proves that the body does not need it, and is over-fed — over-loaded with high protein stuff. Instead of decreasing these poison-producing foods, they are increased — to replace the "loss" — until the patient dies. How tragic to replace waste, while Nature is endeavoring to save you, by removing it!

The next important laboratory test is that of sugar in the urine — Diabetes. The medical dictionary calls it "yet mysterious." Instead of eating natural sweets, which go into the blood, and which can be used — the diabetic patient is fed eggs, meat, bacon, etc., and, in fact, actually starves to death through lack of natural sugar-containing and sugar-producing foods, which have been withheld.

It has long since been proven that all of these blood tests, especially the Wassermann test, are a fallacy.

We, as Naturopaths, cannot ignore Nature's teaching, in any way; even though we may find it difficult to discard old errors hammered into us since childhood.

One of the most misleading errors is the individual naming of all diseases. The name of any disease is not important, and not of any value, whatsoever, when starting a natural cure — especially through fastings and diet. If every disease is caused through foreign matters — and it is — then it is important and necessary, only, to know how great and how much the amount of the patient's encumbrance actually is — how far and how much his system is clogged up by foreign matters, and how much his vitality has become lowered (See Lesson 5 of my "Mucusless Diet Healing System") and, in case of tuberculosis or cancer, if the tissues, themselves, are decomposed. (Pus and germs).

I have had hundreds of cases tell me that every doctor they called upon gave a different diagnosis, and a different name for their trouble. I always surprise them by saying, "I know exactly what you have — through facial diagnosis — and you will see it, yourself, in the "magic mirror," in a few days."

The Experimental Diagnosis

Just as I have already stated in the beginning of this article, you must fast for two or three days. In the case of a fatty type, liquids should be used. The surface of the tongue will clearly indicate the appearance on the inside of the body, and the patient's breath will prove the amount and grade of decomposition. It was even possible to tell the kind of food they preferred most!

Should pain be felt at any one place, during the beginning of the fast, you may be sure that this is a weak point — and the symptom is not sufficiently developed for medical doctors to reveal it, through examination.

Waste will show up in the urine with clouds of mucus, and mucus will be expelled from the nose, throat and lungs. The weaker and more miserable the patient may feel during this fast, the greater is his encumbrance, and the weaker his vitality.

This experimental diagnosis tells you exactly what the trouble is, and how to correct it by starting with a moderate transition diet — or a more radical one — and whether to continue or discontinue the fast.

List of Other Publications

By

PROF. ARNOLD EHRET